HOW TO SELECT AND INSTALL MEDICAL PRACTICE SOFTWARE

HOW TO SELECT AND INSTALL MEDICAL PRACTICE SOFTWARE

1999 Edition

Ronald B. Sterling, CPA

HARCOURT BRACE PROFESSIONAL PUBLISHING

A Division of

Harcourt Brace & Company

SAN DIEGO NEW YORK CHICAGO LONDON

Portions of this work were published in previous editions.

Printed in the United States of America

ISBN: 0-15-606299-2

99 00 01 02 03 EBA 5 4 3 2 1

CONTENTS

PREFACE

This 1999 edition of *How to Select and Install Medical Practice Software* gives medical practices new material to consider when purchasing software, including the following:

- The effect of the Year 2000 Issue on medical practices and on the choice of appropriate software
- The predominance of the Windows operating system
- The cost-effectiveness of electronic medical records
- The possibilities for electronic exchange between the practice and other providers, hospitals, and insurance companies
- What should be included in software and hardware contracts
- Advice on training employees to use medical practice software
- An update of our comprehensive listing of software vendors, including sample prices, features, and other data to help you decide on a vendor that is right for your practice

How to Select and Install Medical Practice Software was written to help medical practices and their advisors focus on key practice management software issues. This book is based on discussions and work with physicians across the country who provide a variety of services under a wide array of healthcare delivery structures. It covers the basic needs of managing a practice's office as well as the utility of various features found in software products. It also explains the mechanics of such emerging areas as managed care, medical records, and electronic exchange of information. Such knowledge will help you not only pick the right system, but also use the system in the most efficient manner. This book is especially useful in its integration of the practice management and patient service side of medicine with the business development and accounting aspects of health care.

For providers, practice managers, and their staffs, this publication is a guide to the processes of selecting and implementing a medical software package and making full use of the system once a decision is made.

For medical consultants, this book pierces the technological complexities to focus on the practical implications of using computers in the medical practice environment.

How to Select and Install Medical Practice Software first reviews recent trends in the medical software industry and gives an informative overview of the medical practice environment. Next, the book walks through the steps involved in selecting and implementing a computer system, followed by separate chapters on general billing requirements, evolving managed care issues, medical records, and electronic data exchange. The later chapters cover key contract issues, implementation steps and strategies, and how to preserve the practice's electronic investment.

Acknowledgments

Any project of this magnitude would not be possible without the contributions of many people. Special thanks are due to Beth Matosko of Sterling Solutions, who advised me on some of the content issues and compiled the list of vendors. Thanks also to Bill Teague and Sharon Odegaard of Harcourt Brace Professional Publishing for their constructive criticism and their on-target advice.

Ronald Sterling
Sterling Solutions
Silver Spring, Maryland

ABOUT THE AUTHOR

Ronald B. Sterling, president of Sterling Solutions, Ltd., Silver Spring, Maryland, is a nationally recognized expert in medical practice management systems, with more than 15 years of experience using technology and information as a competitive weapon. He has worked with numerous PHOs, MSOs, and clinics in 30 states to integrate business options with office automation systems. He has reviewed products from more than 150 healthcare software vendors.

Mr. Sterling is a frequent speaker on medical practice management and hospital-based physician networks to a variety of industry groups. He has presented courses on practice management systems for a wide range of professional and industry groups. In addition, Mr. Sterling has contributed to more than 30 publications, including *AMA News*, *Health Niche Advisor*, *AAOS Bulletin*, *Review of Ophthalmology*, and *Managed Care Report*.

Mr. Sterling earned a BS in Information Systems from the University of Maryland and an MBA in International Business from George Washington University. He is member of the AICPA and the Maryland Association of CPAs.

ABOUT THE COMPUTER DISK

The disk provided with *How to Select and Install Medical Practice Software* contains electronic versions of all the items in the Appendixes, including the chart listing more than 80 medical practice software vendors.

Subject to the conditions in the license agreement and the limited warranty (contained on the disk envelope), you may duplicate the files on this disk, modify them as necessary, and create your own customized versions. Opening the disk envelope and/or using the disk in any way indicates that you accept the terms of the license agreement.

The data disk is intended to be used in conjunction with your word processing software. There are two Windows versions of each document: WordPerfect® 6.0 and Microsoft Word® 6.0 for Windows™. If you do not own either of these programs, your word processing package may be able to convert the documents into a usable format. Check your owner's manual for information on the conversion of documents. The disk is available only in 3.5-inch, high-density format.

Installing the Templates

To install the files on the disk using Windows 3.1, choose File, Run from the Windows Program Manager and type **A:\INSTALL** in the command line or type **A:\INSTALL** at the DOS prompt. You will be asked a series of questions. Read each question carefully and answer as indicated. If you are using Windows 95, select Control Panel from the Start menu. Then choose Add/Remove Programs and select Install.

First, the installation program will ask you to specify which drive you want to install to. You will then be instructed to specify the complete path where you would like the files installed. The installation program will suggest a directory for you, but you can name the directory anything you like. If the directory does not exist, the program will create it for you. The program will automatically install the files in Word and/or WordPerfect subdirectories.

Opening the Files

Open your word processing program. If you are using Microsoft Word or Wordperfect 6.0, choose Open from the File menu. Select the subdirectory that contains the loaded files to list the names of the files. Highlight the name of the file you want to open and click OK or press ENTER. You can also open a document from the File Manager (in Windows 3.1) or in the Explorer (in Windows 95) by highlighting the name of the file you want to use and double-clicking your left mouse button.

The Disk Contents is also available on your disk in a file called "TOC." You can open this file and view it on your screen or print a hard copy to use for reference.

Word Processing Tips

Wherever possible, the text of the documents has been formatted in tables so that you can modify the text without altering the format of the documents. To maneuver within a table, press TAB to move to the next cell, and SHIFT + TAB to move backward one cell. If you want to move to a tab stop within a cell, press CTRL + TAB. For additional tips on working within tables, consult your word processor's manual. It might be helpful to turn on the invisible table lines in Microsoft Word while modifying the document by selecting Gridlines from the Table menu. In WordPerfect, select Reveal Codes from the View menu to reveal all formatting codes at the bottom of the screen; this will help you to determine the shape of the table.

Microsoft Word and WordPerfect are equipped with search capabilities to help you locate specific words or phrases within a document. The Find option listed under the Edit menu performs a search in both Microsoft Word and in Wordperfect 6.0.

Important: When you are finished using a file you will be asked to save it. If you have modified the file, you may want to save the modified file under a different name rather than the name of the original file. (Your word processing program will prompt you for a file name.) This will enable you to reuse the original file without your modifications. If you want to replace the original file with your modified file, save but do not change the name of the file.

Print Troubleshooting

If you are having difficulty printing your document in Microsoft Word or WordPerfect, the following suggestions may correct the problem:

Microsoft Word

- Select Print from the Microsoft Word File menu. Then choose the Printer function.
- Ensure that the correct printer is selected.
- From this window, choose Options.
- In the media box, make sure that the paper size is correct and that the proper paper tray is selected.
- Check your network connections if applicable.
- If you still have trouble printing successfully, it may be because your printer does not recognize the font Times New Roman. At this point, you should change the font of the document to your default font by selecting the document (CTRL + A) and then choosing Font from the Format menu and highlighting the name of the font you normally use. Changing the font of the document may require additional adjustments to the document format, such as margins, tab stops, and table cell

height and width. Select Page Layout from the View menu to view the appearance of the pages before you try to print again.

WordPerfect

- Select Print from the Wordperfect 6.0 File menu. Then choose Select.
- Make sure the correct printer is selected.
- From this menu, press Setup.
- Ensure the correct paper size and paper source have been selected.
- You may be having difficulty because your printer is not compatible with the selected font. You can correct this problem by changing the base font of the document to your default font. From the the Edit menu choose Select All (or press CTRL + A). The entire text of the document should be highlighted. Then choose Font from the Layout menu and highlight the font you normally use. Changing the font of the document may require additional adjustments to the document format, such as margins, tab stops, and table cell height and width. Select Two Page from the View menu to view the appearance of the pages before you try to print again.

DISK CONTENTS

HOW TO SELECT AND INSTALL MEDICAL PRACTICE SOFTWARE

CHAPTER 1 • TRENDS AND STATE OF THE INDUSTRY

CONTENTS

1 TRENDS AND STATE OF THE INDUSTRY

TRENDS

The practice management software industry is subject to the effects of changes taking place in three major areas: technology, the healthcare industry, and practice relationships. Unfortunately, the vast majority of practices do not have the resources or expertise to cope with any one of these issues, let alone with all three at once.

Chances are small that these three issues will resolve themselves in the foreseeable future. Due to the introduction of Windows 98, and the interest of physicians, practices are demanding Windows-based interfaces as a significant item in their product evaluation criteria. The health care industry has yet to settle on business or care delivery models. And relationships among practices and other parties are in a continued state of flux in response to general forces in the marketplace.

In order to confuse practices further, the practice management software vendors are all seeking to capitalize on these opportunities, or, as in many cases, sell out to another company that has a better chance for survival. But for every company that merges (and dozens of mergers have taken place in the past year), a new crop of products appears. Indeed, we are rapidly approaching the availability of more than 2,000 active vendors of practice management systems and almost 1,000 vendors of electronic record systems.

In order to make sense of this, consider the following significant trends.

Windows Systems

With the introduction of Windows 98, we now have seen the third generation of Windows as a major operating system without a significant number of Windows-based practice management products.

Indeed, calls to the major practice management vendors may reveal that their Windows version is not due out for another six months to a year. In fact, in six months from now, the wait may be another six months to a year. Why are so few Windows-based options available?

The bottom line is that the Windows systems must offer significant benefits beyond what is available in the current system in the office. Without a compelling reason to switch to a new product, why should the practice invest the time, money, and effort? Many of the Windows products offered today lack a comprehensive handling of managed care issues and/or have tenuous links to a medical record system. Any practice that is seriously considering a Windows product should be certain of a significant advantage over the existing system before investing.

The Year 2000 Issue

Much has been written about the Year 2000 Issue. Basically, programmers trying to save a couple of characters of space in computer systems wrote their programs to accept, recognize and use only the last two digits of the year on many computer systems. Unfortunately, this means that these programs will incorrectly compute the difference between two dates that span the century mark. In fact, this problem has been around for quite some time. Practices with patients who were born in the previous century have been dealing with this for a number of years.

Practice management software is affected by the Year 2000 Issue in the following three ways:

1. The system may not calculate the correct age of a receivable or the age of a patient.
2. A list of transactions may show an incorrect order. For example, transactions in the year 2000 would precede 1999 transactions in an ascending list by date.
3. Reports and screens may not have space to display the full date; only the last two digits of the year would be displayed.

Some of the problems may be minor irritations (a report incorrectly lists transactions), others may be embarrassing (statements do not correctly age the account), and others could be deadly (a scheduled recall for a patient is not properly managed by the system because the recall option thinks 2/17/00 has already passed).

External Parties and the Year 2000

Even if a practice is 100% compliant, it could still be affected by those it does business with. From the manager of the building to the vendor of medical supplies, one or more of the parties that the practice depends on to keep going could be affected by a Year 2000 glitch. Unfortunately, a practice can do little to compel various parties to prove year 2000 compliance. Also, trying to verify year 2000 compliance among business relationships is beyond the capabilities of the vast majority of practices. Practices may want to consider working together to verify compliance with common business relationships.

In order to provide a minimal level of comfort, ask key business relationships about their situation. Prepare for disruptions to business as the year 2000 approaches. For example, order a larger supply of key items as the end of 1999 approaches. Establish a line of credit to protect the practice from disruptions in payment cycles due to an insurance company problem. The practice should consider the following issues as it prepares for quantifying exposure and mitigating risk of being affected by a Year 2000 Issue:

1. Verify with the landlord that the security systems, climate control, and elevators that service the facility have been tested
2. Verify that the terminals and systems used remotely to access other organizations will work after December 31, 1999. Check the following:
   - Reference laboratories
   - Hospitals
   - Insurance companies
   - Credit card point-of-sale terminals
   - Preferred Provider Organizations
   - Referral Authorization Processors
   - Claims processors
   - Electronic claims clearinghouses
   - Banks (especially lock boxes)
   - Equipment maintenance companies
   - Medical supply distributors
   - Bill printers
   - Collection agencies

To verify the abilities of these parties, send a brief letter inquiring when a version of the system or the software used by the practice to access their system will be available that is year 2000 compliant. If the party's response is less than absolute compliance, consider the effect of a Year 2000 Problem with that party on the practice. If the effect will be substantial, the practice may want to follow up with the party or seek another business relationship.

Internal Equipment and the Year 2000

It is important for the practice not to panic. The first objective is to quantify the nature and scope of the problem. As a practice works towards identifying the problems, it should determine on a case-by-case basis if a problem needs immediate solutions (by December 31, 1999) or whether the practice can live with the problem for a length of time. A practice does have a measure of control over its internal compliance with the Year 2000 Issue. However, it would not be practical to replace all existing equipment by the end of the century.

Note that if equipment is more than a few years old, or if the practice has skipped a couple of upgrades to the system, the practice is definitely at risk. The practice should try to define the problem and develop a rational course of action soon.

In order to quantify the situation, review all existing equipment. Verify that internal equipment will continue to function in an acceptable manner after December 31, 1999. Include the following in the review:

- Lab equipment
- Diagnostic and testing equipment
- Radiology equipment
- Imaging equipment
- FAX machines
- Phone system

The practice should also verify that the office computer systems will work after December 31, 1999. Use the following checklist:

Medical Office Computer System Checklist

The System

____ System startup accepts dates properly.

____ System date rolls over to the year 2000 correctly.

____ Automatic back-up facilities continue to work.

____ Audit trails are properly maintained from 1999 and 2000.

____ Activity dates in the demographic records are correctly managed.

____ Inactive dates after January 1 are correctly managed.

Patient Demographic Information

____ Age is calculated correctly for patients born in the 1900s.

____ Patients are selected based on birthdays that span the century.

____ Medicare eligibility is calculated correctly.

____ Insurance eligibility dates that span the century are managed correctly.

Patient Recalls and Reminders

____ Dates past December 31, 1999 are accepted.

____ Recall reports and letters for future dates into 2000 can be printed.

____ Overdue recalls prior to January 1, 2000 can be tracked.

Patient Scheduling

____ Scheduling templates that are effective into the next century can be managed.

____ Patients can be scheduled into 2000.

____ Appointments are listed correctly in chronological order.

____ Potential appointments in time periods that span the century can be selected.

____ Appointment selection screens correctly move from December, 1999 dates to January, 2000.

Charge Entries

____ Dates of service prior to January 1 are accepted when the system date is past January 1.

____ Service date ranges are accepted that span the century,

____ Insurance information dates (e.g., Date of Injury) for dates of service after December 31, 1999 are accepted.

____ Insurance information dates that span the century (e.g., First Report of Injury in 1999 and last consultation in 2000) are accepted.

Payment Entry

____ Year-2000 payments can be posted to services performed prior to January 1.

____ Unapplied payments and credits from 1999 to year 2000 transactions can be posted.

Billing

____ Statement production past January 1, 2000 can be based on accounts that have not been billed since 1999.

____ Transactions that precede January 1, 2000 are correctly aged.

____ Payment plans and promises to pay can span the century.

Reports

____ Reports can be printed for time periods that span the century.

____ Reports can be printed for time periods in 2000.

Medical Records

____ Treatment plans that span the century are accepted.

____ Chart-tracking information correctly spans the century.

____ Prescription refill logs can span the century.

____ Patient history information correctly handles patients services that span the century.

____ Flow charts can span the century.

____ Lab orders can span the century.

In order to test the system, set the system date ahead to the year 2000 and enter transactions in a test database. If any problems occur, document the problems and notify the vendor immediately.

The legal aspects of the Year 2000 Issue and the lawsuits will be winding their way through the legal system long after the Year 2000 Issue has been solved. Indeed, the first suit against Medical Manager Corporation was filed as this publication went to press.

If a vendor has hundreds or thousands of installations, the vendor will solve the problem in a timely manner. Unfortunately, some vendors will be behind schedule or fail entirely to deal with the problem. Medical offices will run into the problems with the year 2000 as soon as recalls or appointments are scheduled into the next century. Depending on the practice, a solution may be needed very soon. For example, if patients are set up on a one-year recall, the problem needs to be solved by December 31, 1998 so that scheduling can move into the year 2000.)

Practices face two challenges in relying on their vendors to deal with the Year 2000 Issue: vendors must introduce a solution and they must install the solution in their client's offices. In reality, not all vendors will introduce a solution. Indeed, a number of the mergers that have occurred over the past year or two have been driven by the realization that certain vendors couldn't justify development of a Year 2000 solution. The non-compliant vendors sold their installed base of users to another software publisher. Even if a year 2000-compliant version is introduced, the vendor may not have the trainers, installers, and resources to upgrade all of their customers to a year 2000- compliant version. For example, based on one vendor's own representation, it would take 37 months to upgrade all of their users.

In order to find out if a problem exists, contact the vendor and talk to other users. Terms such as "substantially compliant" and "mostly handles the Year 2000" are not a solution. Year 2000 compliance will be needed for everything from demographics to scheduling and billing.

If the vendor is not planning on offering a year 2000-compliant product, or if the solution sounds ineffective, plan a move early to avoid being stuck with outdated software. Vendors are not going to be able to move everyone in time.

If the vendor is planning a move, be careful to insure that the plan is the most effective one for the practice. In fact, some of the upgrades are as costly as getting a new system. Many practices must completely replace their hardware and upgrade their software. Some of these upgrades involve costly conversions of data and retraining of staff. In order to analyze the costs, complete the following chart.

	Year 2000 Upgrade	New System
Hardware		
Software		
Data Conversion		
Training		
TOTAL COST		

If the cost of upgrading is too expensive, the Year 2000 Issue may be the ticket for a new system. When purchasing a new system, make sure that the contract states that the new system is guaranteed to be year 2000-compliant.

Vendors who hedge their commitment may not be the right business partners to resolve this problem and enable a practice to get back to the business of servicing patients.

Software Industry Issues

The continuing problem for practice management software vendors and buyers is the healthcare industry's significant under-investment in technology. Practices invest in information systems at a rate that is one-fourth to one-fifth that of general industry. On the other hand, practices have not found a compelling business or technology justification for dramatic increases in their investment.

The dynamic nature of the healthcare environment and the evolving focus on cost are causing more serious attention to be directed toward tools that can support operations as well as capture more information on patient services and clinical results. A variety of interested parties in addition to providers and practices are focused on capturing information cost-effectively and using the data to control future costs and to monitor performance. Insurance companies are interested in information for disease management, while physician network structures are seeking to establish mechanisms to improve interaction with and among physicians.

For this reason, the healthcare information system industry is attracting a great deal of investor and vendor interest. More sophisticated buyers at the practice level are demanding better information systems that go beyond the traditional patient billing and insurance claim management is accelerating—and product developers are beginning to respond. The evolving needs include the following:

Managed Care

Handling of managed care requirements has been difficult for many vendors because they have attempted to graft managed care needs onto existing fee-for-service data structures. Practices need managed care features to control, monitor, and facilitate compliance with the different terms of each plan. Without these tools to support operations, practices will be unable to cope with the administrative costs of managed care.

Because of the evolving nature of managed care, vendors are continuing to struggle with managed care features. Even most vendors who design products from scratch use the traditional fee-for-service mechanism as the underlying structure of the system. The vendors implement a minimalist handling of referral authorizations and proceed to more advanced capabilities as design and budget allows. Indeed, few products have a report panel that even begins to address the more complex measurement and analysis tools needed in the managed care environment.

Management Analysis

Practices need more sophisticated reporting and tracking structures to manage their own organizations as well as to track performance based on their payor and patient mix.

As organizations add locations and more effectively use their space and personnel, more reporting options and summarization strategies are needed. For example, practices may need to track performance by provider, department, location, and business line.

In the traditional fee-for-service environment, practices measure performance on the basis of realization of charges, and they base compensation on collections by providers. Because of the diversity of arrangements, the management reporting systems must be able to produce comparable reports and to support analysis of an individual practice. Sophisticated practice performance measurements as well as executive information reporting tools are needed to monitor the performance of the complex arrangements that are needed in more complex practice structures.

Products must move from simple transactional reports to management reports. They must also include graphic tools to analyze data in a variety of ways.

Accounting Systems

Existing practice management systems have ignored the handling of accounting issues. Under the current health care environment, more practices need accrual-based accounting procedures and sophisticated tools to measure performance and risk for the larger organization. Such tools will be useful only if they can provide cost analysis as well as payment analysis accounting mechanisms. Larger practices need to be able to monitor profit centers and business lines as well as provider performance.

Products will need to accommodate audit, cost, and reconciliation requirements for more sophisticated business structures. For example, cash management features may be needed for organizations with many sites.

Management of Physician Network and Management Service Organizations

The key to controlling costs is coordinating efforts among a network of providers. Current initiatives seek to offer practices a variety of participation levels and tools. To support these options, products must support sharing of information, facilitating patient services among many providers, and tracking performance across practices.

Products will need innovative data structures that allow for varying levels of services, but they also should produce comparable information for larger practices, Management Service Organizations (MSOs), and physician networks.

These initiatives will include the need to exchange referral authorizations, reports, and, ultimately, clinical information. In order to achieve this objective, organizations will need to communicate with a variety of systems used by other organizations.

Electronic Commerce

Once infrastructures have been established at the practice level, a wide range of electronic data can be exchanged within the health care system. This data exchange would simplify the administration of managed care and would allow systems to highlight problems that are revealed by reports from a variety of sources. For example, the system could identify patients who failed to refill their prescriptions in the pharmacy within the expected time. Similarly, a referral authorization to a specialist could be monitored through the treatment process based on appointment schedules and encounters at the specialist's office.

In addition to sending and receiving information on patient services, an intermediary may be needed to exchange data between different systems.

Health Insurance Portability and Accountability Act

In a few months, the impact of the Health Insurance Portability and Accountability Act of 1996 (H.R. 3103) will start to be felt. The Act establishes a goal to create and implement standards for the "transactions and data elements for such transactions to enable health information to be exchanged electronically." The Act mentions the following transaction types:

- Health claims and encounters
- Health claims attachments
- Enrollment and disenrollment information
- Eligibility information
- Payments and remittances
- Plan premium payments
- First report of injury
- Health claim status
- Referral certification and authorization

Interestingly, the Act seeks to standardize exchanges, such as claims, that are widely available today as well as less commonly used capabilities, such as premium payments and remittances. However, the Act extends exchanges into clinical data through the first report of injury and claim attachments. The electronic exchange of clinical data will present a further challenge to a variety of providers and other healthcare organizations. In essence, the Act gives the industry a not-so-subtle push to establish and implement electronic exchanges that will allow everyone to improve efficiency and effectiveness with the right management tools and computer systems. The Act will also increase the volume of electronic traffic and speed the deployment of electronic data exchange infrastructures, such as the Internet, intranets, and traditional communication server technologies.

Although the timetable in the Act may not be met, the Act raises the level of functionality and sophistication that practices and others will need as the exchanges mentioned in the Act become reality. Addressing these issues will give providers a compelling reason to move from their legacy products to tools and vendors that can make a bottom-line contribution to patient service, provider productivity, and practice management, as well as meet the connectivity requirements of the act.

Point of Care/Service and Medical Records

Medical records and point of care/service pose the most challenging aspect of computers in practices. To date, the use of electronic medical records is spotty. For example, +MEDIC has offered Autochart for several years, but only 5% of practices that use +MEDIC products have bought this particular product.

The use of effective electronic medical records requires agreement on what information is significant, a standard way to collect that information, and a mechanism to deliver information. These requirements demand that computing resources be deployed more extensively; they also require providers to rethink their acquisition and use of electronic medical records.

Providers are just starting to recognize the challenges of implementing these tools in a useful manner.

The practice management software industry is subject to the continuing challenges of significant changes in healthcare as well as the continuing evolution of the computer industry. Dramatic changes in the functional needs of practices have posed a particular challenge to vendors. Many vendors are far behind in developing modules that address managed care issues effectively and support evolving practice business models. Practices are having a difficult time articulating their needs and directing their efforts towards meeting requirements that are constantly changing.

The following trends are worth keeping an eye on:

- **Features and function sets** Electronic data exchanges and core business needs will force vendors to offer as standard features items that are considered progressive today (e.g., referral authorizations). Therefore, features such as treatment plan management, capitation accounting, patient flow management, and truly integrated medical records will differentiate products in the future.
- **Replacement of legacy systems** A wide range of legacy system vendors will not be able to enhance their products to keep up with future practice needs or Year 2000 requirements. Any consideration of product purchases should include the ability and willingness of the

vendor to meet these evolving requirements. If a vendor has not established a vision and acted to offer such products, that vendor will not be a viable player, regardless of its ability to meet the current needs of the practice. Many products are still focused on the insurance claim process. The products that will be successful in the future will have to address clinical issues as well as electronic data exchanges (e.g., referrals and injury reporting). Many of the data structures and audit trails currently used by a wide range of vendors will not easily accommodate these requirements.

- **Integrated delivery systems and provider network management** To date, many vendors have only scratched the surface of the transactions and product features that will be needed to facilitate working relationships in provider networks and integrated delivery systems. A wide range of new data and features will be needed to rationalize relationships and improve operational and clinical efficiency in the healthcare industry.

In the absence of a dominant business and patient delivery mechanism, these challenges will continue to test practices as well as vendors for the foreseeable future. However, increasing numbers of practices are recognizing that they need to have an effective information system to meet the needs of the evolving healthcare marketplace. Awareness of these needs and awareness of the value of having a wide range of patient information that currently is neither accessible through computers nor tracked by the practices will result in additional investments to meet the demands of the evolving marketplace.

STATE OF THE INDUSTRY

Over the last few years, the acquisition of practice management software vendors has continued. Regional players have been acquired by national firms. Several smaller vendors have also acquired complementary technology to enhance their product line. For example, +MEDIC acquired Compudata of Atlanta, Georgia, and CBSI of Rockville, Maryland. Both CBSI and Compudata offered practice management systems that needed dramatic changes to meet managed care issues and take advantage of new technologies. +MEDIC was attracted to these companies by their strong installed base in key markets. Similarly, InfoCure of Atlanta is buying up small regional companies to build a critical mass of installations to catch the eye of investors on Wall Street.

Unfortunately, the acquisition strategy does not always pay off. The recent problems experienced by PCN Health Network may be related to acquisitions that in reality did not fit a strategic need in the market.

This activity will continue. The vendors with large installed bases are continuing to look for next-generation products that will improve the lot of their current users. Some vendors with legacy technologies and smaller installed bases are looking to sell their installed base to a larger vendor with the critical mass of users that can justify development in Windows, as well as the extensive changes needed to accommodate managed care and integrate with medical record tools. And all of these vendors are competing for a decreasing number of buyers due to merger and acquisition activities among practices.

To protect their investment and position, practices that are acquiring systems must be careful to examine and verify the vendor's ability to stay competitive and its desire to remain independent. In the absence of either indicator, practices should be wary of committing to a software publisher that is positioning for a sellout. Failure to develop progressive solutions and cuts in research and development are early warning signs that the vendor may not be committed to a long-term presence or is pumping up performance before sale.

However, for each software acquisition, another couple of new players spring onto the scene. Larger software vendors, as well as small start-ups, are taking a new look at this evolving marketplace. The key opportunity that practice management systems represent is an underserved market and a legacy technology base. Indeed, the deployment of PCs in many practices has resulted in a substantial base of underused workstations.

The practice management software industry is being challenged by the continuing changes to the business models and operational methods used by medical practices and by the evolving healthcare environment. From the development and evolution of integrated delivery systems to the latest permutation of "managed care," the industry currently is attempting to respond to permanent changes while trying to finesse its way through changes that are perceived as temporary.

These conditions will continue to challenge buyers and sellers of practice management systems. The current status and long-term viability of the large number of existing healthcare information system vendors should be a major evaluation criteria for a practice considering an investment on its information system technology base. On the other hand, practices will have to increase their information system budgets dramatically to meet their business and patient service needs.

Such investments will position the practice to provide more added-value benefits to patients, insurers, and employers.

CHAPTER 2 • OVERVIEW OF THE MEDICAL SOFTWARE INDUSTRY

CONTENTS

2 OVERVIEW OF THE MEDICAL SOFTWARE INDUSTRY

With more than 1,800 active practice management software vendors and 800 electronic medical record publishers, the medical software industry is one of the most fragmented software market segments in the United States. The entire medical practice software industry has revenues of approximately $4 billion per year.

Software companies range from those that have a few products installed locally to those that have thousands installed nationally. Local or regional software publishers may have a few employees who must fill many roles, or they may employ 50 or more people divided into functional departments. National firms may employ hundreds of development, support, and sales personnel.

A number of national firms distribute their products through other companies in selected cities. Some vendors have a hundred or more distributors while others have a few relationships. Indeed, a medical practice seeking to purchase practice management software may find several vendors of the same product in a single area, as well as identical products sold under a variety of product names. For example, there are private label versions of Practice Partner, Medical Manager, and PCN Health Network. Private labels are used to differentiate the same product being distributed by several sources; yet the different names give the impression that there are a variety of packages.

INDUSTRY BUSINESS MODELS

Practice management software vendors fall into two basic business models: direct sales organizations and distributor organizations:

Direct sales organizations Direct sales organizations offer one-stop, single-source shopping for hardware, software, training, and support from a single location, regional locations, and/or local offices. Indeed, some vendors have gone through several cycles of establishing local offices and then closing local offices to centralize operations until the next iteration. Some vendors supplement a single central office with small sales offices in strategic locations. Most local and regional software publishers, as well as publishers of several nationally distributed products, use the direct sales model. IDX, +MEDIC, and Reynolds and Reynolds are examples of direct sales organizations.

Distributor-based organizations Distributor-based organizations offer their products through independent sales and service firms. The initial contact for the sale, installation, and support of the product will be between the practice and the distributor. Typically, the practice will have a sales agreement with the distributor as well as a separate software license from the publisher of the software. Medical Manager, PCN Health Network, Physician Office Manager from HBOC, and Practice Partner are examples of software products that are sold primarily through distributors.

Each of these business models has a direct impact on support and flexibility of the medical practice's use of the system.

Support

Direct sales organizations can maintain a standard of support for all their installations. Conversely, the quality of support from a distribution sales organization will rest primarily with the distributor; the original publisher simply sells the product to the distributor, who resells the product to the medical practice. The level of service and support can vary dramatically from one distributor to another. Because of the increasing complexity of a medical practice's operations and the functional sophistication of the leading software products, publishers are taking a greater interest in the business and medical practice skills of their distributors. Indeed, dissatisfaction with a product can be attributed to a failure in support as much as to a fundamental flaw with the practice management system. Therefore, anyone charged with choosing a medical software package must be careful to pick a distributor that can support the practice.

On the other hand, under a distribution situation, the practice may be able to call upon several support and sales options to compete for its business or replace its current distributor if it becomes dissatisfied with the support and service it is receiving.

Flexibility

Direct sales organizations typically are not as flexible as distributors. Even though standard capabilities are important for support, direct sales organizations usually have more stringent contracts and stricter rules about how they do business and what hardware they will support. The larger organizations want to limit the number of variables they have to deal with when supporting a site. Therefore, many direct sales groups require certain hardware setups and frown on medical practices purchasing their own hardware. Standardized hardware setups eliminate a number of support variables for a company that is trying to support many users across a wide geographic area.

Such standards also affect the support and installation effort. Direct sales organizations are more consistent in their level of support and in the quality of their final product. Choosing a distributor must include carefully examining the quality of the equipment, the support staff, and the services offered. Even though distributors generally offer greater flexibility, the practice could end up having the only installation of its kind in the distributor's customer base. For example, the practice may prefer one brand of printer over the brands supported and sold by the distributor. The distributor, however, may not be aware of the special drivers and commands needed to allow optimal use of that printer with the software.

PRACTICE MANAGEMENT SOFTWARE INDUSTRY CHALLENGES

As a practical matter, a number of software products handle patient billing and insurance claims management quite competently. Indeed, software publishers have been working for more than two decades on refining these capabilities. However, these old product standards will not keep a company competitive.

The consolidation of healthcare providers is having an impact on the practice management software industry and all other businesses that serve these providers. As practices consolidate, there are fewer potential users of a software system. If 10 sole practitioners join forces, chances are that eventually a single software vendor will serve them. The combined practice will have more sophisticated needs and will demand a product that will meet future needs as well as keep up with current requirements.

Products that offer traditional PMS features are meeting only the minimal requirements of these more sophisticated business structures.

The most serious challenges facing practice management software vendors today are (a) the impact of managed care on practices, (b) the evolution of electronic data interchange relationships between practices and other healthcare providers, and (c) the need to establish a quick and easy way to record and access patients' clinical information. These evolving needs are taxing the strongest of the software publishers. To meet these challenges and maintain a viable product in the marketplace, vendors are employing a variety of strategies.

Continuing Independent Development

As a result of dramatic changes in healthcare management systems, a whole new class of management tools is needed. A number of vendors are attempting to address these needs independently.

In some cases, vendors "work around" the ability of their existing system to handle a new requirement. For example, basic work-arounds in products designed for fee-for-service may not maintain an audit trail of the "value" of services provided in a managed care program, or they may not measure obligations for future services. The practice may need to know the cost of future services for existing conditions. Adding viable ways of tracking evolving constructs and maintaining appropriate audit trails requires a great deal of time and effort, and not all organizations have the wherewithal to support such development. Some organizations may also be reluctant to make dramatic changes when legacy systems—existing systems in their customer base—will complicate implementation or conversion to structures that will handle new industry requirements more effectively.

Combining Forces with Other Vendors

A flurry of acquisitions and pseudo-acquisitions, such as co-marketing or joint development projects, by practice management software vendors has been occurring for several years. The larger software vendors are seeking to establish a greater presence in the industry and gain installed bases in areas where they are weak. It is interesting that each of the major hospital software vendors has acquired a practice management vendor or has established a strategic relationship with one.

The smaller regional players have an interest in working with a larger group, because of the high cost of adding capabilities to handle the evolving medical practice's needs. From a marketing perspective, the larger provider groups are closely examining the viability of the software vendors with whom they work.

If a software vendor is acquired by another company, only one of the products will survive over the long term. It is not economically feasible for a software publisher to maintain two products targeted to the same market that have the same capabilities. At some point, the software publisher will choose to commit new development to one product and maintain the second product at a minimal level.

Establishing Links to Other Products

As a stopgap measure, many software vendors are establishing links or relationships with add-on products that fill the gaps in their existing product lines. For example, several vendors are using MedicaLogic, a medical records package, and EZ-CAP, a claims tracking tool for managed care environments, in place of adding a medical records system or creating functions to manage referrals in a managed care environment.

These arm's-length working relationships offer vendors and users a quick solution. The implications of such a move, however, can be extremely important. Specifically, is the relationship a long-term strategic one or a temporary fix to a product deficiency? In either case, the connections between these systems and the practice management data may be tenuous or subject to timing differences. For example, how will the demographic information shared by the two products remain the same? Depending on the connection, the practice could be subject to data integrity, timing, or audit problems.

If a vendor uses more than one product, the user should be sure that the connections between the two products meet the needs of the practice. If the two products do not "talk" to each other, will the practice have to collect information manually from the two systems to complete key management reports? It is especially important to ensure that the links between the basic practice management system and the medical records or managed care system can be audited and verified for accuracy and integrity.

Unfortunately, vendors as well as providers are trying to deal with moving targets in healthcare and technology. The medical industry is undergoing significant changes as new healthcare delivery models evolve, and providers must develop working relationships with a variety of organizations. For example, whole blocks of existing patients may move to a new plan that uses a combination of fee-for-service and capitated carveouts (e.g., basic care or specific procedures) based on various service needs. These hybrid plans may include unique setups and classification structures.

The computer industry must cope with product life cycles that are measured in months. For example, even though Windows 98 has just been released, many practice management vendors are still developing their first Windows product.

THE PRACTICE VIEW

As a result of the evolution of the medical industry in general and of medical practices in particular, medical practices face serious challenges on a number of fronts. First, the administrative burden on practices has been growing and is becoming more complicated in managed care environments. In general, more than 70% of nonprovider expenses are costs for people and space. Furthermore, it has been estimated that from the scheduling clerk to the provider, everyone spends 25%–40% of his or her time searching for information or recording information. The average practice

Figure 1: Basic Medical Practice Flow

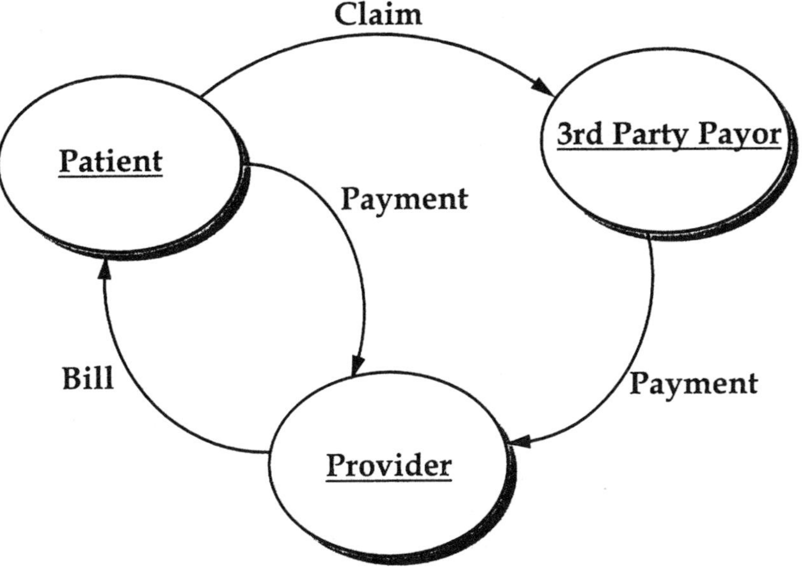

Figure 2: Basic Patient Service Process

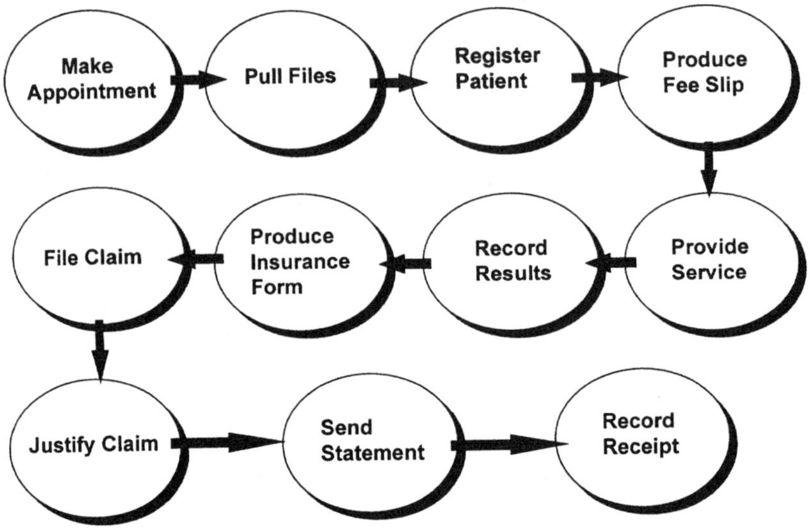

touches paper 22 times to complete the entire patient service process for a single encounter.

Figure 1 shows the general flow of information among the practice, the patient, and the third-party payor. Figure 2 illustrates the internal practice flow needed to support the basic process in Figure 1. Note that many of those steps may be repeated several times or may require several actions for a single service for one patient. A patient can change appointments several times. The recording of results may include a brief provider note at the time of service, compilation of a more extensive note at the end of the day, and final transcription and editing of the formal treatment note the next day. Many practices have even more intensive paper-processing problems.

To survive in the managed care environment, providers are exploring or are being lobbied to join forces with other providers in a variety of structures. The general trend is for practices to increase in size to achieve economies of scale. Some of these initiatives involve the acquisition or merger of various practices; others allow providers to join in a loose coalition to share management and business services.

These evolving business and patient care models are accentuating the need for new computerized tools to go beyond the traditional patient billing and claim collection tools. These functional areas include the following:

- **Managed care** Managed care encompasses a variety of management and operational support features to facilitate movement of patients and compliance with individual contracts that the practice enters into. Chapter 5 reviews this area in detail.
- **Management reporting** Management reporting includes more sophisticated reports that address tracking of more complex business and patient structures. For example, practices with multiple locations

and a range of services may need to manage and track performance by location as well as by revenues and charges related to business lines (ex. Therapy, Ambulatory Surgical Center, Medical Services). However, these reporting requirements also include tools that support "What if?" analysis and measuring results based on a variety of metrics. Management reports are reviewed in each section.

- **Electronic commerce** In addition to the widely available electronic claims and evolution of electronic remittance, there is a variety of information that would dramatically improve efficiency and service. For example, primary care providers who can identify patients who have stopped taking their prescribed drugs or who have not taken advantage of certain wellness services will be better prepared to initiate actions that increase compliance and ultimately control costs. Electronic commerce and EDI issues are discussed in Chapter 7.
- **Accounting systems** Larger practices and more complex business structures need more effective accounting tools that go beyond the needs of the traditional cash basis medical practice. Chapter 8 reviews the accounting issues and needs.
- **Large practice and physician network management** Many of the items mentioned throughout this book are related to managing practices of all sizes. However, a variety of these items become more significant and important for larger practices.
- **Point of service/care and medical records** Medical records are a very hot topic. Everyone is talking about them, and many providers want them. Medical records pose a serious challenge to software vendors and providers. Software vendors must develop products that maintain adequate connections among the medical records, plan-specific care standards, and the financially oriented information on a patient. Providers must change their behavior to take advantage of medical records, and invest a significant amount of time to properly implement and deploy medical record tools. Chapter 6 covers medical records issues.

From more sophisticated accounting skills to better marketing and patient service strategies, practices need better tools to adequately meet the requirements of health plans and the expectations of patients.

The literature on these movements in the healthcare market is wide-ranging. In spite of the differences of opinion on the delivery models and structures, it is universally recognized that effective technology tools are the key to achieving success in the evolving healthcare market.

CHAPTER 3 • THE SELECTION PROCESS

CONTENTS

3 THE SELECTION PROCESS

The key to any practice computerization effort is the criteria that are used to select the medical software. A variety of methods can be used to determine if a particular practice management system meets a practice's specific requirements. Measuring a potential system solution against an incomplete list of requirements will doom the entire project to failure.

To establish the correct selection criteria, a number of different key issues and requirements must be considered. Unfortunately, many practices focus on the biggest problem of the day. For example, one practice was primarily interested in a more attractive bill for its patients, while the system it had been using produced only a basic balance forward bill that did not support complex insurance claims. Seeking primarily to produce a more attractive bill, the practice did not think to include in its selection criteria the ability to document issues as it worked with insurance companies. The billing questions affected three staff members, but the insurance billing problem affected more than ten staff members.

In many cases, practices find it especially difficult to conceptualize the functions needed to deal with emerging issues when the basic needs of the practice cannot be met. Nonetheless, computer system implementation is so expensive and has an impact on so many people that the practice should not plan to use a system for only a few years. Even stopgap computerization measures must consider current problems as well as expected needs. Indeed, selection criteria should include issues that are expected to affect the practice for the next few years. For example, a practice that will be opening up a new office next to a same-day surgery center should include location-based profit tracking and scheduling in its selection criteria. The practice may also need to consider inventory and surgical tracking requirements to support the surgery center. Practices in areas with low managed care penetration should plan on handling a greater managed care volume in the future.

In some cases, the computerization process will necessitate a complete overhaul of the practice's policies and procedures. Ideally, the practice will invest the time to consider the optimal way to operate. Although the current flow of patients and paperwork should be considered, it should not be the basis for new methods; the current methods should not be automatically moved to the new system. The optimal method is one that has been closely reviewed, scrutinized, and tested to insure that the practice meets operational and patient service needs while taking practical advantage of investments in technology.

In reality, a variety of products can meet the needs of basic patient billing and insurance claims. The greatest added value of any system, however, is how that system helps staff and providers serve patients and manage the practice. Regardless of the size and complexity of the practice, the evaluation effort should yield a concise list of key relevant differences. With this information, the practice can make the final decision based on the relevant issues and not get sidetracked by issues that do not affect the practice or are already adequately handled. For example, a primary care provider may skip features needed by specialists.

RESOURCES FOR SELECTING A COMPUTER SYSTEM

Selecting and implementing a new computer system will take a great deal of time and effort, during which the practice must still follow its daily routine. Who will choose and implement a new system is a key question facing many medical practices. A variety of tasks must be performed that require a range of skills and knowledge. It might be true that, given enough time, almost anyone on the staff could select a good system and make the right choices about how to use it. Unfortunately, few staff members will have the necessary time.

Some practices spend six months or longer looking at various systems, without ever arriving at a decision. To use everyone's time most effectively, the practice should consider resources that could supplement internal capabilities and put the effort on a fast track. Outside resources are most useful for tasks that require specific knowledge and will be needed only temporarily. For example, outside resources could be used to evaluate a system's ability to meet the needs of a practice and to negotiate a contract. Inside resources should be relied on to develop detailed procedures after the operational strategy has been defined. Outside resources may be effective at facilitating the implementation process, but internal resources should redesign the forms and compose the collection letters. By using outside resources for guidance and specialized skills, the practice will give its own staff the greatest exposure to the selection and implementation processes. The knowledge the staff gains will stay with the practice after the project is completed.

Outside resources include CPAs, consultants, trainers, and installers, and may be available from an accounting firm, a healthcare consulting company, or a systems integrator. Depending on capabilities within the practice, outside resources can be used in the following ways:

1. **To develop an information technology strategy** To establish an appropriate measurement tool for any new system, a strategic information plan would define the role of computers in the practice. An outside resource will bring fresh options for the practice to consider.
2. **To facilitate compilation of a requirements list** The list should consider current and future needs of the practice. It would downplay generally available capabilities but should include critical capabilities

and deficiencies of the current system. The list should include patient service needs, managed care issues, and management requirements. An outside resource could work with the practice's staff and management to help the practice develop a targeted list.

3. **To compile a request for proposal to distribute to appropriate vendors** The request for proposal will address functional issues as well as business requirements.
4. **To evaluate vendor proposals** An experienced consultant will be able to analyze vendor proposals effectively. Those knowledgeable in practice management systems will be able to comment on a vendor's representations.
5. **To negotiate a contract with the vendor** Negotiations will focus on contract terms, services, and the implementation schedule to structure a results-oriented relationship with the vendor for the initial effort as well as for future support.
6. **To develop an implementation plan to manage and guide the project** The plan would include specific responsibilities and due dates.
7. **To design implementation strategies or customized features** An outside resource can help analyze and select the software features and operational options that will be most appropriate for the practice. The outside consultant can also help a practice navigate through the system setup and implementation efforts.
8. **To develop a conversion methodology to move data from the existing system to the new system** The conversion strategy would document changes to existing codes as well as the use of new fields in the new system.

There are other areas in which outside resources may help the practice. In any event, the practice must gather all of the resources needed to establish the computer system and use it effectively. Failure to do so will affect the practice every time a patient is served.

KEY STRATEGIC ISSUES

Before undertaking any system evaluation process, a practice must decide on any strategic business or computer system issues. Strategic issues should address the long-term needs of the practice. Some of the more serious strategic issues to consider are the following:

- Hospital connectivity
- Affiliation with a medical network
- Adding a new office
- Increasing the number of providers
- Increasing services

Hospital Connectivity

Practices that have a close relationship with a hospital should consider hospital connectivity strategies. Some hospitals are closely associated with a practice management system that is used in its clinics or promoted by the management service organization (MSO). Other hospitals do not use a particular all-inclusive practice management product but use a hospital management system that has a practice management module.

The practice should not follow the hospital strategy without looking at other options, but if all other considerations are equal, the hospital connection may be a deciding factor. The system that is connected to the hospital-sponsored physician network or physician–hospital network will allow the practice to work with the various providers for referrals and general relationships. On the basis of such considerations as access to electronic mail and other electronic information (e.g., referrals and images), the software will have to be the designated package or will have to be able to operate within the connections provided by the hospital. If the hospital system is not appropriate for the practice or will not support certain key requirements, the practice should avoid the product regardless of hospital support.

Practices should consider the long-term effects of committing to the hospital's connectivity strategy. Practices that are affiliated with several hospitals may want to avoid purchasing a system through one hospital and limiting their options with the other hospitals. On the other hand, practices that are affiliated with only one hospital may derive greater benefits and a better working relationship by committing fully to the hospital's connectivity strategy.

For more information on the types of connectivity and the different organizations that offer connectivity options to practices, see Chapter 7, "Electronic Data Interchange."

Medical Network

Similar to its connection with a hospital, the practice may be affiliated with one or more independent provider networks. These networks typically include a credentialing process and a third-party payment and authorization (TPA) process.

A practice must maintain appropriate credentials for each provider as well as meet the specific reporting requirements of each plan. As the number of physicians and the number of contracts grow, the time and expense of maintaining and reporting information multiples. Education, certification, insurance, and licensing information must be maintained for each provider. The system should allow for user-defined reports for the credentialing information.

The TPA process includes the traditional claims adjudication process as well as referral and authorizations management. If the practice management software does not work with the TPA management system, the practice may have to enter information in more than one place to maintain the managed care relationship. For example, the office of a specialist may have to record a service associated with a referral into its practice management system and then use a different terminal to record the service in the TPA system. This lack of connectivity may make it more difficult and expensive to serve other providers in the network.

TPA systems must track the specific terms and conditions of each plan as well as the services a provider is contracted for by plan. The TPA system should manage a claims adjudication process that is sensitive to the specific issues of each plan.

Adding a New Office

In most medical software packages, adding offices has a greater effect on the setup of a system than on the selection of one. However, some products cannot accommodate multiple offices or produce relevant productivity and management reports for each office. The report selection criteria should include office locations and should allow the practice to review provider activity across offices.

In order to support multiple offices, the software should also offer audit trails to track activity and security to limit access by location. The system should offer balancing reports with detailed or summary information by location, operator, transaction type, and day. Closing procedures should allow offices to be on different closing cycles. For example, a remote office may close several days after the office that is next to the billing operation. An operation with many offices may need batching features to control transactions from many locations.

For managing many offices within a practice, a variety of strategies are available, some of which will limit flexibility and patient service options. One key area is appointment scheduling. Many systems require a separate "appointment book" for each provider and location combination. For example, one appointment book would exist for Doctor A in Office 1 and another appointment book would be kept for the same doctor in Office 2. The office staff must check two places to schedule an appointment for a patient, and the doctor will receive two schedules, one for each office. Ideally, the system should allow identification of the location of the doctor within the schedule. For example, the provider can be assigned to Office 1 in the morning and Office 2 in the afternoon.

Some systems do not allow multiple offices to be managed in a single database. Conceptually, a database is a file drawer that contains all the information for an office or a practice. If each office has a separate database, a common set of procedure codes, diagnostic codes, and other key codes must be set up. Otherwise, each office could develop a different file setup, and the reports would be difficult to compare. Office procedures must be identical if they are to produce easily comparable reports. For example, if some offices date receipts on the day payment is received and others use the date on the check (the date the patient or insurer sent the check), the daily reports would not reflect the same activity for each office.

Increasing the Number of Providers

If the practice expects to dramatically increase the number of providers, various management and reporting issues should be closely explored. Depending on the size of the practice, the system should accommodate departments, provider-level service profiles, and scheduling for a larger number of providers. Some scheduling systems limit the number of providers that may be displayed on a screen at one time, while other schedulers do not support the selection of providers by offered services. For example, a large practice may need to determine quickly whether a service can be offered in-house rather than through an outpatient referral; the proper system can help control outside referrals and costs.

If the practice has many providers, software should allow the staff to evaluate providers in several different ways. For example, the software should be capable of grouping providers as primary care physicians or specialists, as partners or non-partners.

Increasing Services

Practices that expect to add services should consider how to manage or track those new services. For example, a family practice may add group counseling sessions. The scheduling for group counseling differs from standard patient scheduling. An orthopedist may add a physical therapy service or a return-to-work program. Treatment and patient management issues for these services would differ from those of a surgical orthopedic practice.

Some larger practices may plan to offer more comprehensive service and geographic coverage to make themselves more attractive to managed care plans. A close look at the service's planned offering will help ensure that the system that is selected and set up actually supports those efforts.

To compile a list of relevant issues, the practice will have to undertake a strategic review of the various contingencies and changes expected over the life of the system. Certainly there will be unexpected changes, but the practice should not select a system without considering expected changes. Indeed, several system selection efforts have failed to consider pending mergers and have resulted in wasted efforts and lost investments.

COMPILING A LIST

In order to evaluate a software system, the practice will need selection criteria that are relevant to its particular situation. Before such a list is compiled, it may be helpful for everyone in the practice to participate in filling out a Basic Practice Assessment. (See Appendix 1 for a sample.) The basic assessment will yield a top-level profile of the practice to guide its efforts. Any serious problems should be noted and should serve as checkpoints throughout the selection and implementation processes. If specific aspects of the current system are particularly useful, these items should be documented and the evaluation process should seek them in the new system. It should never be assumed that a newer system will improve upon features that may be taken for granted in the current system.

A number of methods—for example, functional lists, scenarios, and acid tests—can be used individually or in combination to compile the list. Chapters 4–8 review specific areas and present a variety of issues to consider.

Functional Lists

Functional lists itemize the specific detailed needs of the practice. Often these are combinations of the various lists drawn up by each staff member. A functional list could include specific items (e.g., the system should be able to print bills in ZIP code order) as well as general issues (e.g., the system should be easy to use). See Appendix 2 for an example of a functional list.

Although functional lists are easy for everyone to understand, they do not necessarily reconcile competing requirements. A requirement in one area may peripherally affect another group of requirements. For example, a staff member may want to use an in-house alias to call up a procedure, but management wants procedure analysis in a sort order that would not be supported by the in-house alias.

Scenarios

Scenarios describe sequences of events and tasks that occur or should occur in any practice. Scenarios specify not particular items but a flow of processing and information. A sample scenario might read:

> Can assign messages to users, providers, and patient accounts to log future activities. Users can establish action items for the future or record a significant event. Each message is tagged with author, type (e.g., billing or patient treatment), and date information (e.g., sending, tickler, resolution). The system can display worklists of pending messages by user or by message type. Uncleared messages with tickler dates continue to appear until resolved.

Specific functional requirements or practice issues can also be included in the description. Scenarios can be compiled easily in a review of current procedures; those current procedures should be adjusted for any known problems as the scenarios are created.

Acid Tests

An acid test consists of a concise set of issues related to a specific area. As many areas as necessary—appointment scheduling, office routing, and managed care, for example—may be itemized. Figure 3 offers one example.

Figure 3: Acid Test—Office Routing

KEY ISSUE:
Can patient flow be managed/monitored ?

EFFICIENCY:
Are various records for an encounter connected?

FUNCTION:
Are office routing results recorded in the schedule?

OFFICE ROUTING:
Are patients checked into the office and department?

PATIENT SERVICE:
Can wait times be analyzed ?

PATIENT MANAGEMENT:
Can treatment trigger recalls or treatment steps?

Note that the acid test considers the effect of the processing on other areas in the practice. Each question is formulated to identify key processing requirements keeping in mind the need for efficiency, functionality, office routing, patient service, and practice management needs.

SELECTING CANDIDATES

To select a system properly, a practice must determine the scope of its needs and must manage its expectations. Practice management systems come in a variety of structures at a variety of costs. With dozens of products to choose from, one could spend a long time trying to review each option thoroughly. As a practical matter, the practice will want to focus its efforts on a limited number of candidates.

To quickly narrow the field to a few contenders, some "show-stopper" issues should be considered:

Does the hardware platform fit the strategic vision of the practice?

Some practices limit their search to software packages with a large number of existing installations. However, some of these products are at the end of their life cycle. Indeed, some of the established products are based on exotic hardware or systems that are no longer competitive in the marketplace. For example, a practice that is using an old operating system may be limited to an inadequate word processor for transcription; or a practice may be left stranded when support for its hardware setup is eliminated because there are few users in the area.

Is the vendor strong enough to succeed in a more demanding environment?

As noted earlier, medical practices need more sophisticated tools to manage an ever-more-demanding business and service environment. To succeed in this market, vendors need the ideas to solve the problem, the will to implement the solution, and the dollars to finance the changes. Unfortunately, even some large companies lack the will or the ideas to meet the evolving needs.

Software publishers and their staff may be unable to abandon old methods in favor of more effective tools—because of their fear of the new products not being accepted, or because their knowledge base does not fit the new needs. In order to survive, software publishers will have to be financially stable in order to invest in continually upgrading their products and improving the levels of expertise and service they offer to users. If a vendor does not have the financial strength to fund development, the package it offers may not keep up with the emerging needs of its customers.

Can the vendor support the practice?

No matter how good the package is, the key to success or failure is support. Good support is particularly important to medical practices, because few practices have internal support people. If a vendor does not have local users or a viable support mechanism, the practice should consider other options. If there are no local users, the practice should make sure—for example, by checking references the vendor provides of existing users with remote support—the vendor has served other practices effectively in a similar situation.

Does the product handle key requirements?

In compiling its list of requirements, the practice may have identified a number of items that are absolutely necessary. Those items should be presented to the vendor up front and a demonstration requested of the software's ability to handle them.

Is a comparable practice using the product?

The vendor should be able to offer the name of a client, preferably local, that has a comparable operation and installation. It is especially important to verify that the comparable practice is being *served* by the same organization that is trying to sell the system, not just using the same system, and that the providers have fully implemented the system.

Is the product within the budget established by the practice?

A computer system will surely be the biggest administrative expense a practice will ever undertake. There are numerous systems, costs, and options to consider in the process of selection and system design. However, a reasonable estimate can be calculated for budget purposes before a new system is sought. The following scheme gives a general idea of the necessary financial commitment. This estimate will provide a rough idea of the level of commitment an organization must make. Note that there are a variety of decisions that can significantly affect the final cost.

In general, a billing and scheduling system will require one or two terminals per provider at a cost of $4,000 to $6,000 per terminal. Medical records costs far exceed the cost of billing systems since providers need access to the medical records from anywhere in the facility. An additional investment should be made to insure availability of the system. (The practice may be able to get by for a few hours with a billing system outage, but it is inconvenient and inefficient for providers to see patients while the medical records system is inactive.) Medical record expenses can range from $25,000 to $50,000 per provider.

These estimates understate the costs for practices that have extensive communication needs across many offices. Practices that use a separate corporation for a few providers or serve several practices also will incur additional costs for each practice. More specialized software, such as radiology management systems and occupational health management tools, will cost more than the estimate given above.

THE SEARCH

There are several different ways to seek out the right product. Some practices will rely exclusively on contacts with colleagues, others will assign various staff people to seek out choices, and others will read ads.

Regardless of the method chosen, the list of requirements is the touchstone throughout the evaluation process. In order to proceed with the quest, the practice may choose to identify key vendors and call them in for a demonstration, or may undertake a formal request for proposal process.

The Demonstration

If the decision is made *not* to develop a request for proposal, the practice may proceed directly to the demonstration process. The demonstration should be a formal exercise, with staff using their list of specific items to grade each product consistently and being especially careful to focus on the items that are particularly important to the practice.

The Request for Proposal

The request for proposal (RFP) is a document that defines what the practice is looking for. It is a communication tool that formally establishes a wide range of parameters about the practice's expectations of the product and vendor.

The RFP can be quite extensive, or very brief. In some larger organizations, an RFP is an absolute necessity, because of the size of the project and/or procurement requirements. Even if an RFP is not required, the practice may want to consider formulating one, since an RFP helps organize individual users' thoughts and the selection process as a whole. This factor may be especially important for those who do not regularly engage in software evaluation and system selection.

In any event, the RFP would include one or more of the following sections:

- **Introduction to the organization** Many RFPs introduce the organization and explain the organizational structure, mission, and objectives. The Introduction may present a history of how the entity was formed as well as a discussion of any predecessor organizations. The Introduction may also explain the current technology base, as well as the expectation of using existing equipment or converting existing data to the new system.
- **Objective for the project** The strategic and tactical objectives for the project are explained and discussed. Objectives can include adding capacity and managing new processes, as well as supporting new initiatives. Some proposals explain the urgency of moving forward to resolve specific problems with the current system.
- **Explanation of the process** The proposal may present a specific schedule for completing the selection and implementation process. The various tasks may include:
  — Receipt of letters from vendors about their intentions
  — Due dates for final questions
  — Visit to the site(s)
  — Receipt of the proposal
  — Completion of the evaluation
  — Demonstration of the product
  — Notification of the winner
- **Terms and conditions** The RFP may itemize specific contract terms and conditions that are needed. See Chapter 10.
- **Specific items** The list of items that are needed would be included in the RFP. Vendors will have to comment on their ability to meet the

requirements using the existing system, with future enhancements, or with some customization work.

- **Vendor responsibilities** The RFP should specify the specific work items the vendor will have to fulfill.
- **Proposal format** The RFP may specify the format of the vendor's proposal. The proposal may include the following sections:
  — Introduction to the vendor
  — List of specific items with responses
  — Cost proposal for the software, hardware, and services

The proposal is the formal response to the RFP from each vendor. Some groups even provide a disk with the RFP to help the vendor respond with a properly formatted list of specific items. After receiving the proposals, the evaluation staff will review them and grade the ability of each vendor to respond to the specific needs and to meet expectations within any cost limitations.

Any vendors that pass the proposal and evaluation process should be brought in to demonstrate their product and discuss in detail the specifics of system implementation as well as the contract terms.

EVALUATING SYSTEMS

One of the larger challenges is to decide whether a system *meets* a requirement. Meeting any specific need is frequently a subjective issue. As systems are reviewed in light of the needs of the practice, the system's ability to handle each requirement should be scored. Before formal evaluations are made, it may be helpful to try a few demonstrations to become accustomed to reviewing products.

Before the evaluation, specific requirements should be presented to the vendor's representative so he or she can prepare setups or samples. The demonstration will be more focused and effective if examples are used that relate to the specific needs of the practice.

During the presentation and evaluation of a system, each item on the list of specific requirements could be marked as follows:

0—Not Available
1—Unacceptable
2—Meets Requirement
3—Meets Requirement Well
4—Exceptional Capabilities for Requirement

Notes should be kept on aspects of the system that are poor or exceptional, on odd work-arounds, and on issues that do not make sense. Such notes will be a key tool in making a final decision and presenting final concerns to the favored vendor.

It is probably most efficient to limit the number of people who participate in the evaluation to a few key players who are familiar with the operation and the requirements list. When the choices have been narrowed to one or two, the system can be demonstrated to the entire staff.

CHAPTER 4 • SELECTION CRITERIA

CONTENTS

4 SELECTION CRITERIA

When a medical practice selects a software system, literally hundreds of issues should be considered. A number of issues will determine priorities, including service philosophy, target market, and payor mix. Some important items are available generally. For example, a wide range of products can perform basic patient billing and insurance claims tasks. Other items may be more difficult to locate. For example, anesthesiology billing uses a complex calculation to adjust charges according to the number of patients seen at one time. Furthermore, many systems lack an on-line collections tool.

ISSUES TO CONSIDER

This chapter reviews selection issues for the practice to consider in compiling its list of requirements.

Practice Size

Growth in practice size and in patient flows challenges the standard organizational rules and structures. Larger organizations need a variety of profit center tracking, departmental management, and regional organizational structures. They also need stronger audit tools to verify that employees are coding transactions correctly and entering relevant information.

In order to produce audit reports that are needed to monitor activities in several locations, transactions should be tagged with the operator, location, and date of entry. Transactional reports by location, operator, provider, and date can be used to verify and audit activities. For a practice with a large number of sites, reports should include those that support auditing of an operator as well as a roll-up report to verify transactions by user group or department as well as by location. The auditability of the data is a critical item for organizations with multiple locations and operating units.

Larger organizations manage a larger number of master file entries. A single provider may use 100 to 150 procedure codes, while a large multispecialty practice may use 1000 codes or more. Be careful to insure that systems can handle the number of records needed for the practice size. For example, some systems are limited to 10 providers while other allow 100 or more. Because of turnover in staff and physicians, leave adequate room to track active as well as previously active providers.

Provider, referring physician, procedure code, and diagnostic code files should track codes by category (e.g., referring practice, area of medicine), as well as present detailed analysis of activities. The practice will be able to monitor activities at a manageable summary level (e.g., area of practice) and delve into the details (e.g., by procedure code) as needed.

The transaction files should store information for an extended period of time. Being able to track trends, performance, and treatment standards over a fairly long time will provide the practice with invaluable insights into service and risk issues. Unfortunately, many systems have file size limitations that would require key records to be purged. Other systems lack the trend and management reports to analyze performance over time. In either case, the practice would be unable to derive the benefits of longer-term recordkeeping.

System Structure

Each computer software product is built on a data structure that determines how information will be processed and accessed. The system structure also determines the ability of a feature or function to meet the needs of the user. When the practice is considering a particular feature, the level of the system that the feature addresses should be reviewed.

Medical practice software can control features at a number of levels: the system, the practice, the provider, the location, the account, the patient, or the transaction. The level at which an item is controlled will determine how flexible the system is. Flexibility can vary from product to product. For example, some products assign diagnoses at the patient level. When charges are entered, a diagnosis must be picked from the patient's record, or the diagnosis must be changed in the patient's record. Practices that treat patients for a particular problem may prefer standard diagnoses at the patient level. Similarly, some systems allow patients to use an insurance company from the guarantor file only. A child of divorced parents who is covered by insurance from both parents would be difficult for such a system to handle.

Be certain to check the "level" at which various items are managed in the current system. An attractive data item or feature may prove useless to the practice if it cannot be managed at the right level. For example, a case record used to group procedures that use the same insurance claim details may not be an effective tool to track case payments or costs.

Open Item Accounting

Open item accounting is particularly significant to medical practices. Practice management systems produce analytical and management reports from the underlying financial transactions. If the system does not exactly match the insurance payments with the specific procedure code, the practice cannot verify the insurance coverage or review the specific payment without retrieving the original explanation of benefits (EOB) form.

Lacking a matching payment, the system will be able to produce only general realization reports. For example, the system may be able to report on the percentage collected from an insurance company for all submitted charges, but it could not tell that 100% of lab charges were paid while office visits were subject to many write-offs. Procedure-level analysis can help verify payments, identify problem charges, and analyze the patient service mix.

Several open item methods are available in practice management systems, including encounter-level open item, procedure-level open item with balance, and procedure-level open item with transactions.

Encounter-Level Open Item

The encounter-level open item method posts payments to the encounter. All procedures under the encounter are kept for reference and claim-filing purposes. The transaction register will display the encounter. The charges and payments that were applied to the encounter can be reviewed.

Encounter-level open item does not match payments and adjustments to specific procedures, so management reports based on encounter-level open item cannot be used to analyze procedure-level information. Because procedure-level approved amounts are not tracked in the system, office staff must verify the approved amounts and payments from each insurance company manually.

To work around these limitations, some vendors recommend that only one charge be entered for each encounter, so that all payments are posted to individual charges. If a separate encounter is entered for each procedure, open item at the procedure code level can be maintained. The audit trails may be obscured, however, and there will be multiple encounters for a single patient visit and/or charge ticket. More important, insurance claims may become confused, because a separate claim may be filed for each encounter in the system.

Procedure-Level Open Item with Balance

In the procedure-level open item with balance method, payments are posted to the specific procedure and the system maintains a running balance for each charge—for example, a $50 charge has a current balance of $10. The payment record includes the amount posted to charges and the original amount of the payment—for example, $20 of a $30 check was posted to procedures and $10 is tracked as an unapplied payment. The transaction register displays the original charge and the remaining balance for each procedure.

Such systems can calculate realization for the practice at the procedure level. The realization reports by procedure code will correctly reflect both the total charges and the dollars received for those charges. However, this method does not preserve the details of how the procedure charge was paid or adjusted. The practice could not produce a detailed procedure analysis by insurance company. The practice would have to review the original EOB manually to compile information on receipts by insurer or to compile the details of a particular insurance payment.

Procedure-Level Open Item with Transactions

The procedure-level open item with transactions method is similar to procedure-level open item with balance, except that posting records are written in a cross-index file for each payment or adjustment for each procedure. The transaction ledgers display the payments and charges, and the posting details for each procedure, charge, or adjustment can also be viewed. The specific charges and adjustments that were posted to a procedure can be reviewed, as well as the charges that were affected by a payment or adjustment. This permits a review of the specific application of each financial transaction.

This method maintains a complete record of financial activity, but it requires more work to post payments and adjustments to accounts. The increased posting effort will virtually eliminate the need to pick up the EOB again, since the payment details are kept in the computer.

Electronic EOBs can make open item posting with transactions less of a problem for the practice. The computer will automatically post the payment at the procedure code level on the basis of electronic posting information obtained from the insurer.

Ease of Use

Anyone who buys a computer system must consider the practical issues involved in actually using the system every day. The key issue for daily use is the ease with which a user can access the system and get work done. If a system is very simple, but users must constantly resort to handwritten notes and hard copy records to fulfill basic requirements, the system is not easy to use. On the other hand, a system that does everything but uses obscure codes and screen-thrashing (i.e., requires multiple screens to do a basic task) may be comprehensive but not easy to use.

Regardless of the system, new users will need 3–6 months of experience on the system before they really understand it. Ease of use on the system requires balancing the needs of the practice with the effort required to get the job done.

Users have different opinions about what makes a system easy to use. Some like graphical user interfaces (e.g., Macintosh and Windows) better than character-based systems (e.g., DOS, UNIX). Indeed, some users like Macintosh systems better than Windows-based systems, while others prefer UNIX character-based systems over mainframe character-based systems. Such preferences depend on the background and experiences of each user.

The following guidelines should be considered in determining a system's ease of use:

1. **Mobility** It should be possible to navigate quickly from one function to another. For example, in a sequence of events dealing with a patient, what has to be done to post a charge, calculate the patient's balances, post a payment, and schedule an appointment? What happens if the user stops the process to check another patient's status and then tries to return to the first patient's file?

2. **Help** System help includes selecting codes from various files as well as on-line instructions. For any prompt that is connected to a file, the system should easily help the user look up the relevant code and fill the field. On-line instructions should include easy-to-understand labels and access to instructions.

   Help files consist of specific help areas maintained by the system as well as areas for notes and comments. Be certain that the practice can record nuances of the various parties the organization must cope with in the system. For example, attach information on specific pre-authorization procedures for an insurance plan or list important contacts at other medical practices.

   Larger organizations should consider establishing help files that provide information to users on practice policies and procedures on-line. That way the staff members will have access to the latest information and not be using an old copy of procedures, price lists, and checklists. Be careful to insure that custom help instructions will survive through system upgrades. Some vendors will allow a practice to change their help files but will overwrite the changes in the next release.

3. **Screen layouts** The screens should be consistent in presentation and operation. Products that use different labels for the same field on different screens or that jump around among the screens for data entry may be more difficult to learn and use. Commands to initiate a particular activity should be consistent throughout the system. Otherwise, users will have to remember where to enter an "M" for modify versus a "C" for change.

Security

Smaller practices have a limited number of employees who enter information and a small number of terminals, so security generally is not a serious issue. Larger practices, on the other hand, have a variety of security issues to deal with. For example, practices that operate out of more than one office must establish controls over charge entry and payment posting to ensure that each site properly audits and verifies daily activity.

Note that some practices maintain a back office collection and billing unit that enters all charges and payments. The back office operation must maintain appropriate tracking of all transaction batches by location to ensure that the documentation trail from the site to the billing office to the computer system is preserved.

The software should limit access at the functional level, meaning that most employees can schedule appointments but not post charges. Additionally, the system should support audit trails over changes to transactions and activity reports by user and by date; in this way the practice can audit the activity of a particular user. Audit reports and daily reports should include an option to print transactions for a specific posting date as well as date of service. The posting date is the date the transaction is entered into the system; the transaction date is the date the service was performed or the payment received.

A more important problem is limiting access to medical records. Electronic medical records may help providers access information on a patient. However, electronic records must be protected to prevent unauthorized changes and unauthorized access. Once a medical record has been verified, the system should prevent changes by any user. Access should be controlled through a number of options, including limiting access by type of medical information and by patient. General office staff could be given access to a patient's medical record summary sheet but little else. Nurses could have access to prescription information but be prevented from accessing information on special patients. For example, access to the medical records of a famous person may be limited to the provider.

In some practices, employees at a particular site have access only to the records of patients served by that site. In other cases, employees can access information for only a particular provider's patients.

Regardless of the access security maintained over patient look-up, charge entry, and medical records, many systems allow users to print information on reports for patients they could not access interactively. For example, a user may be limited to working with patients for Provider C but could produce a report for Providers A through F. This flaw may be addressed by limiting report production to a few supervisors, although this may not prove practical for certain practices.

It should be possible to print different audit reports to analyze activity and changes in order to support security efforts. Bad tagging of transactions or lack of audit trails over changes will limit ability to monitor activities and verify enforcement of practice guidelines and procedures. For example, systems that allow users to tag transactions with any audit code may not offer adequate tracing information. Products that offer audit reports by user for a range of dates and transaction types will satisfy many verification needs.

One way to secure data is to have a separate database for each security group. Many systems allow the user to define separate files of information for a separate business or corporation. Most of these systems do not even share CPT or diagnostic codes between databases, so a user on one database cannot move easily to another database without another set of security codes. The separate databases complicate the reporting of aggregate information across many databases. The system must be programmed to allow summarization across databases that use different coding systems.

Another issue to note is that the vendor may require a practice to buy a separate user license for access into each database. For example, three back office employees may need access to four databases. Depending on operating procedures, the practice may have to buy 12 licenses for those three employees.

Patient Scheduling

The key benefit of patient scheduling is being able to document the entire patient service process. From the time a patient calls the office for an appointment until the final bill is settled and recalls are established, a variety of patient and practice management objectives can be addressed. Documenting this process allows the practice to monitor quality and performance standards.

When the patient calls for an appointment, an automated system can help the scheduler do the following:

1. **Address the patient's scheduling needs.** Patients have a variety of scheduling needs that can be fulfilled through the computer. Automated scheduling manages the flow of patients through the office, so that office staff can take the time to register patients properly, verify information, and note any issues or concerns. The information can be printed on the router to notify the provider of any special needs at the time of service. Similarly, the schedule could be used as a trigger for marketing or patient information efforts. For example, new patients could be sent a welcome packet and test information could be mailed to patients who schedule a test.
2. **Manage the flow of patients' services.** Computerized scheduling allows for optimal provider scheduling. Each provider can set up appointment scheduling templates that make the best use of his or her time or that balance various existing obligations with time to see patients who have new problems. The flow of patient scheduling may be an indicator of practice performance and future services. For example, if all of the consultation slots are not filled for a provider, the volume of procedures may drop four to six weeks in the future.
3. **Verify insurance benefits and authorizations.** Staff can verify patients' insurance information when scheduling appointments. Under managed care plans, the user could ensure that an appropriate referral authorization is available for the appointment. If a referral has expired, the practice could arrange to obtain one before the appointment occurs. Ideally, the system should allow a staff member or physician to associate an appointment with a treatment plan, recall, and/or referral. The connection can clearly be seen between services and care obligations.
4. **Solicit payment commitments.** When the patient calls, the practice could review the account and address any collection issues. Payment commitments could be noted in the appointment record for follow-up by the check-in clerk before the appointment.

Some patient scheduling systems may require information that a patient does not know or that only a medical technician can properly record. For example, some schedules accept a diagnosis and CPT code. Unless a patient was under a treatment plan, that information could not be determined. Others use volume and resource management based on a specific procedure and the average service time. One practice, for example, scheduled new-patient appointments in 30-minute slots and allocated treatment appointments 10 minutes each. As a practical matter, most practices use less specific scheduling methods (e.g., one patient every so many minutes).

Another practice had all the patients arrive on the hour. Patients would have to wait to register with the receptionist as well as wait for the provider. Patient scheduling has a direct impact on service, collectibility, and productivity.

One way to support efficient and responsive scheduling is to use appointment templates by provider. An appointment template allows staff to schedule according to the type of appointment, frequency, and a standard time span. Each provider can have his or her own template. A typical schedule template defines specific appointment slots for a standard provider day, being as specific or as general as desired. A pediatrician may wish to see a patient every 10 minutes, while an orthopedist may see new cases on the hour and follow-up cases every 10 minutes from the half hour to the hour. Some practices can even schedule by procedure code.

To schedule an appointment, the system should display the relevant day and move easily forward or backward in time. Staff should be able to select the time quickly and record the information. Typically, the appointment is associated with an appointment code, a length of time, and a free-form note. Once entered, the appointment can be moved to another day and time or removed from the schedule with a few keystrokes.

Appointments related to a pending treatment plan should be connected to the plan. The practice will be able to check off each treatment step as it is completed and thereby identify patients who have dropped out of treatment plans.

When an appointment is scheduled, the operator should be presented with a variety of service options:

1. **Display the patient's financial status.** The patient's financial and demographic information should be directly accessible from the scheduler. The operator can then easily answer questions about the account or address an insurance matter, as well as verify the patient's information and update critical information. Flag follow-up tasks as well as standard procedures. For example, insurance may be verified every six months through a tickler or note.
2. **Produce a letter.** If a new patient is being served, the operator may want to produce a welcoming letter. Or, depending on the type of appointment, the practice can automatically send a letter of instructions. For example, a patient who will be seeing a gastroenterologist may need to be told to follow a restricted diet for 24 hours before the visit. The system should maintain a record of the correspondence with the patient.
3. **Leave a note for the physician.** The staff user should be able to associate a note with the appointment or leave a note for the physician.

Appointment Disposition

The system should track appointment activity. If a patient is seen, a report of appointments scheduled, without charges, will facilitate daily audits. If a patient did not show up or canceled an appointment, the system should record the disposition of the appointment. Then, the scheduler could review the frequency of a patient's no-shows and cancellations when allocating future appointment time to that patient. The practice may choose to save choice appointment slots for patients who regularly keep their appointments and to work in unreliable patients if they do show up.

Appointment disposition also documents patient-related disruptions to meeting quality objectives or patient treatment plans. For example, the system could alert the provider that a patient who requires periodic testing has failed to make or keep several appointments.

Some systems keep only summaries of appointment dispositions, while others tag the appointment status on the original appointment record. A summary consists of a count of missed appointments that the system maintains as cancellations are recorded. When the information is kept on the original record, the operator may review the specific purpose of the canceled visit and the reason for the cancellation. When the disposition information comes from the appointment records, the appointment records should be kept on the system until the cancellation information is no longer important.

Be careful to insure that the practice is not burdened with old appointments records. For example, some products display all of the appointment records in chronological order. Therefore, the user would have to pass through all of the old patient appointments on the system before getting to the latest records.

Physician Scheduling

In multi-office and hospital-based practices, the scheduling of physicians and support staff can be time-consuming and costly. The costs include patient service missteps as well as paying a provider to cover extra time or hiring another provider to fill the missed assignments. Computer-based scheduling may offer a cost-effective management tool to help larger, multi-specialty practices and primary care groups with specialties cover their patient service responsibilities adequately.

Provider scheduling tools allow a set of rules and requirements to be defined. The practice may have certain specialty coverage requirements as well as various coverage rules. A hospital-based radiology group may provide fluoroscopy and computer-assisted tomography (CAT) services 24 hours a day. The applicable rules, which include various partnership issues (e.g., vacation, weekend coverage), hospital rules (e.g., subspecialities), and guidelines (e.g., consecutive working hours), can often be difficult to manage and administer.

Most of these products are expensive due to the complex programming rules needed to maintain appropriate coverage and track workloads.

As a practical matter, many practices resort to a spreadsheet and try to review the schedule manually for compliance. Other practices use customized applications based on general database programs.

With a custom application, be careful to insure that all of the coverage parameters that are significant for the practice are included. Such information would need to include provider- specific credential and specialty information.

Patient Information

The patient is the central contact point for access to and use of information. Because the patient is the recipient of medical services, all information is connected to the patient's record. Typically, a guarantor—parent, spouse, employer, attorney—is responsible for the patient's charges. Attorney guarantors are common in personal injury and worker's compensation cases. Employer guarantors are common for industrial medicine or executive health services.

Guarantors

Systems track patients through a guarantor or allow a guarantor to be assigned to a patient. When the patient is tracked through the guarantor, the guarantor is entered as a master account and the patients are entered under an account number with a suffix (e.g., 1234.01). This strategy limits the number of patients who may be assigned to a guarantor and allows for only a single guarantor for each patient. Limits on the number of patients per guarantor vary from six patients to 99. This limit will easily accommodate families, but it may not be sufficient for employer and attorney guarantors. If patients are covered by other guarantors, insure that all of the patients connect to a single account. Ideally, an unlimited number of patients should be able to be connected to a guarantor.

When a patient changes guarantors or is treated for services covered by another guarantor (e.g., industrial medical clinic treatments and drug testing), a separate patient record must be created for the patient's charges covered by the second guarantor. Each patient account is linked to a separate guarantor account and can maintain insurer information for the separate account. Charges, notes, and medical records are posted to the separate patient account.

Such systems will produce a separate form or document for each account when various reports are produced. In essence, the system maintains two relationships with the same patient. One of the patient records will only reveal the services provided to the patient under the relevant guarantor. Remember to look under both accounts to gain a complete picture of patient service. Indeed, the patient will be counted as two patients on management reports. Some systems link the separate patient account to a master patient record. With such a system, all the accounts for a specific patient can be accessed from a single master patient account.

A few systems allow for multiple guarantors for a patient. The guarantor may be assigned to the case or medical problem record. Each patient's account is linked to a separate guarantor account and can maintain insurer information for the separate account. Charges, notes, and medical records are posted to the separate patient account. The provider must examine both accounts to gain a full understanding of the patient's situation. Some systems link the separate patient account to a master patient record. With such a system, all the accounts for a specific patient can be accessed from a single master patient account.

Any of these guarantor structures can be used effectively, depending on the type of practice. Practices that must frequently track multiple-guarantor relationships for a single patient would benefit from systems that allow for multiple guarantors. Other practices would be able to use either approach.

In any event, make certain that the guarantor feature is backed up by on-line and billing features that will smooth the workload. The system should allow for review all of the accounts under a guarantor. Billing options should include transactions tagged with the patient name as well as separate pages for each patient.

Demographic Information

Each patient record is associated with demographic information that profiles the patient for the practice. Analyzing demographic information can help a practice monitor its performance and service opportunities. For example, age distribution can help a pediatrician identify targets for marketing programs. Specific demographic information on patients is discussed in the following paragraphs.

Employment

Employment information is essential primarily for practices that work with insurance companies, but it can also be a valuable resource for identifying marketing opportunities—for example, some practices provide employee wellness seminars—and assisting in collections on problem accounts.

If employer information is not linked to a master file, the employment information will have limited use. Users cannot be depended on to enter a particular employer the same way each time. For example, employees may not include the complete name of the company, omitting an initial "The," or they may use an abbreviation, such as "BCBS" for Blue Cross and Blue Shield.

Insurance

Insurance company information is used primarily to file insurance claims. In many systems, only the name of the insurance company is tracked and coded to the patient. Due to the plethora of plans and the increasing importance of tracking the terms and conditions of active plans and insurers, the practice may need more information about these plans. At a minimum, providers should track the fees paid by key insurers and verify insurance payments. Practices need to log the expected payment and other key terms for the top plans used by patients.

Plan information includes the covered services, physician participation and, in some cases, locations. If plans are tracked, be sure to summarize plans by insurer. Management report by carriers across plans will allow evaluation of the complete relationship with the payor. Similarly, plans can be put into categories (e.g., capitation, case, contract) to evaluate the performance of various types. For example, reduced fee contracts may be losing money for the practice because the standard fee schedules are discounted too much.

Plan-specific information also drives how the system processes covered charges. For example, a practice may participate in an independent practice association (IPA) plan sponsored by an insurer but not in the fee-for-service plan of that same insurer. The practice would write off the difference between the payment and the charge for the IPA plan but promote the fee-for-service bill to the patient after the insurance company has paid.

Account and Patient Classifications

Many practices deal with several thousand patients for each provider. Classification codes place patients in logical groups for processing, management, reporting, and other purposes. Codes can also drive fees, billing, letters, and, even appointment scheduling.

Patients can be classified by a grouping (e.g., good payors vs. bad payors), by practice relationship (e.g., relative of long-time patient), by collection status (e.g., account is delinquent or is with a collection agency), or by a variety of other classifications. The practice could even classify patients by the reason they gave for leaving the practice (e.g., moved, practice too expensive, found a better practice) or joining it (e.g., practice highly recommended, part of employer health plan).

The more classifications one patient has, the more accurate the records will be. Avoid systems that offer only one or two status codes that are used for many purposes. It may be too difficult to track patients in all the different ways that are relevant to the practice.

Patient History

Many practice management systems encourage the purging of information shortly after a bill is completely paid. However, much of this information has enduring value for a variety of purposes. With it, providers can review historical information quickly to find patients who were provided certain services or to review the business relationship between the practice and a patient. In offices that use transcription or electronic medical records, users can access and review information without having to retrieve paper records.

The computer system should have the capacity and tools to research the details of a patient's billing and treatment history. The system should be able to store large amounts of data for reporting and analysis without impeding regular processing. For example, some systems present only lists of transactions in sequence by date, requiring the user to pass through all of the old records before reviewing current information.

On-line users should be able to view transactions by type (payment, charge, adjustment), date, and related transactions, as well as viewing all of the adjustments and payments applied to a charge.

Preauthorization

Providers must get authorization from insurance companies to treat continuing problems or provide certain services. The authorization number the insurance company provides should be noted, along with the contact's name and any notes on various terms.

All insurance details—including preauthorization information—should be easily associated with charges at the time of charge entry. Insurance details include claim information as well as comments, the insurance adjuster, description of the problem, and dated notes to document the history case.

Some systems allow for cases that define a variety of filing and treatment information for a continuing problem. When entering an encounter that is related to the case, the user tags the charge with the case code; then all of the insurance details will be associated with the charge and vice versa. Claim management will be easier, and the practice can review all charges for a particular case on one report.

Hospitalization

Tracking and logging patients' hospitalizations allows the practice to monitor utilization and to ensure that charges have been correctly posted. Hospital service records are difficult to control and log, because the provider is serving patients away from the practice and therefore without the support of the practice's administrative staff. Hospital information is becoming more important for several reasons. For example, managed care requires more coordination to insure that all of the providers have proper authorization and the number of locations that many doctors work out of is actually increasing with the expansion of ambulatory surgical centers.

Hospitalization information includes the facility, treatment, and location of the patient. Hospital tracking modules produce route forms that the provider can use to record services, instructions, and follow-up information.

Some products also manage surgical scheduling requirements.

Treatment Plan

Treatment plans document the services to be provided at one or more future encounters that have specific dates or delay times between steps—for example, an ongoing therapy program or a series of tests to monitor a condition. As services are provided, they would be checked off on the treatment plan; the computer could also identify treatment plans that have not been completed within the recommended time. Some practices have quite formal sequences; others are less formal. Each treatment plan step can be associated with a scheduled date or delay, a procedure code, a note, and a flag on the disposition of the treatment.

Treatment plans have always been used by doctors. However, few doctors document the plans in the patient records. By documenting the treatment plan in the computer, office staff can easily coordinate treatments plans with patient appointments and identify patients who have dropped out of the treatment process.

Notes

In a medical practice, notes and comments are important to each functional area (e.g., billing, patient, treatment). If a system has noting capabilities, the practice can record the note and make important information on the patient available to all users. Notes can document a complex family situation, a patient's preferences, or administrative issues. Practices could also use notes to document discussions with an insurer or other party.

Some systems provide a single note field that works much like a continuous word processing file. With such a system, however, the user would have to scan the entire file to find a particular bit of information, and related notes may be mixed in with other issues and comments. The ideal noting function should code the note with an issue or reference code (e.g., insurance, complaint) and tag the note with the user and date. Then all notes can be searched on the basis of specified criteria. Some systems also allow the user to enter a follow-up date that can act as a tickler.

A limited number of systems can attach a note to a financial transaction on a patient's record. For example, a note explaining the insurance company's payment could be attached to the payment record and printed on the next billing statement.

User-Defined Fields

User-defined fields can store specific information about the practice without customization costs. User-defined fields may be associated with the guarantor, patient, charge, appointment, and payment records.

Most systems allow a label of defined length for an alphanumeric field. Some products have fields with various characteristics. For example, one system allows a screen with several date, numeric, and alphanumeric fields for which the user can define the field labels. Other systems allow the user to determine the label, length, and characteristics of the user-defined fields. Some provide for reports that allow selection of patients by user-defined field.

User-defined fields can store information that the standard system cannot, for example, a key date, information on the patient for case retrieval, or additional patient classifications. Note that many medical records are composed of user-defined fields. Selected medical record profile information could be stored in user-defined fields.

The key feature that makes user-defined fields valuable is the reports, which can be generated by selecting patients with certain values in a user-defined field. To take full advantage of reporting, be sure that the system supports consistent use and coding of user-defined fields.

OFFICE ROUTING

Most medical practice software systems will produce a router or fee slip on an ad hoc basis or for all appointments scheduled for the day. The practice uses a list of the scheduled appointments in an appointment book format to check off patients as they are seen. A separate appointment list by provider, time, patient's name, and appointment type should be used to serve the needs of multiple staff members.

Patient Flow

As an office increases the number of patients it serves, paper-based appointment strategies can no longer track patient flow efficiently or keep everyone in the office informed of the patients remaining to be seen. Instead, the computer system could be used to manage this flow of patients.

Tracking patients through the office can be as simple as logging in their arrival and departure times, or the practice can log patients as they move from the waiting room to the examination room to the laboratory and so on. The office routing data could be used to monitor quality and to audit patients' charge entries. For example, patients who were checked into the lab should have a lab charge on their bill.

Patient flow tracking can be a natural by-product of the treatment process. As a provider calls up information on a patient, or a technician records procedures, the patient could be checked into each location. Systems that track patient flow allow the user to display the active patients by department or arrival time or other criteria. The practice's staff can check on a patient's status, and management can monitor patient flow. For example, a work list of the patients in the lab could be used to select the next patient to be served. Nursing staff could review the patient check-in information to select the next patient to be escorted to the examination room or to review patients in the waiting room. Otherwise, the staff must constantly phone the nurses' stations to let them know a patient is waiting in the front check-in area, or the nurse must watch continuously for arrivals.

Patient flow tracking will help the medical practice manage resources more effectively and analyze patient flow patterns and wait times. Flow information could be used to alert staff about patients who may have been kept waiting an excessive amount of time or to adjust staffing to improve patient flow. The statistical information also could be used to monitor waiting time and visit time as measures of the quality of care. The various results and time analyses could be used to encourage staff and to document performance to insurers.

Route Slips

Route slips are used to record services to patients and the patient's condition at the time of service. Many practices use the route slip as the patient's receipt at the completion of the visit. The route slip is presented at checkout, and the clerk calculates the total charge and records any payments on the route slip.

Typically, a clerk enters the information on the office copy of the completed form into the computer system or passes it to a back office operation for posting of the charges and payments. These methods were derived from traditional batch systems. However, the practice should consider real time entry of patients' charges at checkout or even during the service process.

When a patient checks out, the staff member could enter the charges from the route slip and the computer could calculate the amount due. Ideally, the system would calculate the estimated amount of the patient's responsibility and display the amounts for the checkout clerk. This way, the checkout clerk can clarify the estimated payment and the patient's obligations at the time of service.

Another option is to collect charge information as the patient is treated. Each provider or technician would post charges to the system as part of the service process. The charge posting process may be connected to the medical records or to a lab information system.

Posting the charges when the patient checks out or as the patient is being seen will improve information flow within the office. However, it should be easy to enter in the information as the patient is served. In these situations, the computer system must be flexible and easy to use for both clinicians and administrative staff.

Charge Coding

Posting charges is challenging because of the complexity of procedure and diagnosis coding. There are two coding standards: current procedural terminology (CPT) codes and *International Classification of Diseases*, 9th Revision (ICD-9), codes. CPT codes describe the type of services (e.g., brief office visit, stress test) provided to a patient. ICD-9 codes identify why the services were provided (e.g., patient has diabetes). Both coding standards are changed to accommodate new procedures and finer distinctions of problems.

The combination of CPT and ICD-9 codes also affects payments made by insurance companies. A misleading combination (e.g., chest X-rays for a kidney stone diagnosis) will result in rejection of the claim and additional work for the practice. Most practices commonly use 75 to 125 CPT codes and hundreds of ICD-9 codes. Depending on the practice, these codes may be assigned by the provider, a nurse, a technician, or a billing clerk.

CPT codes are further affected by modifiers that describe the specifics of the service and that can inflate or deflate the approved amount. For example, an assisting physician uses a modifier to indicate that the provider was not the primary surgeon on a job. Another modifier indicates that a second surgical procedure was provided during the same operation as another procedure. In both cases, the modifier will deflate the amount that the insurance company will approve for the physician who performed the work

A variety of coding tools may be used to help providers and their staff code charges. Some systems include coding tools that the practice maintains, while other systems have a working relationship with third-party coding programs.

Coding tools that come with software systems include tables that connect CPT and ICD-9 codes. Allowed and disallowed coding combinations can be set up. If a user attempts to enter a code that is not allowed, the system will display a message. Lists of allowed diagnoses are sometimes used to speed charge entry. For example, after the user has entered a CPT code, a list of common diagnoses may be displayed.

Codes can also be deactivated. Because codes can be changed, a flag in the master record will block further use of the code yet allow previous charges with that code to be kept in the system and management reports to remain useful. Systems that do not have deactivation flags typically require deletion of codes from the master file after all transactions with the code have been purged.

Some products allow for look-up of codes for any word in the description. A user looking for a code for a chest problem would be presented with "Chest Pain" or "Pain, Chest." Most systems search only from the beginning of the description.

Although these tools are useful, maintaining coding tables and cross-reference tables can be time-consuming and difficult. When the practice uses a new code, it will have to be added to the cross-reference tables. Further, all of the cross-references will have to evaluated when codes change.

Third-party automated coding tools help the user identify the appropriate code. A number of practice management system vendors offer working relationships with these products. Basically, the operator hits a function key to leave the practice management system and invoke the coding software. The coding software includes look-up and elimination tools to select the right code. Once the code is selected, the operator returns to the practice's product, and the code is automatically inserted in the appropriate field.

For CPT code selection, the operator can select codes on the basis of combinations of words, or can "drill down" through the codes (i.e., search for more and more specific service codes). These products can also inform the user of new codes that have replaced old ones. The user can review the specific definition of the code or the standard services that are provided with the code.

ICD-9 coding is more complicated. In addition to providing the tools for CPT codes, ICD-9 coding systems include questions with which to fine-tune coding at the right level. ICD-9 codes include various levels; depending on the conditions related to the diagnosis, the user must code at a different level. For example, some diagnoses codes use two additional digits to specify a body part. The ICD-9 coding software will ask specific questions, depending on the diagnosis, to select the right level of detail and the appropriate code.

BILLING

Many systems limit when and how patients can be billed. Depending on the patient population and payor mix, many practices need more than one billing format and a variety of patient and insurance company billing mechanisms. Yet, the billing system must allow for clear and effective communication with patients. Older patients, for example, may be confused by a detailed bill of the various adjustments, contract writedowns, and payments for Medicare services. A simpler bill may ease such patients' anxiety and speed up the receipt of payments. Several managed care organizations have special billing formats and coding systems.

Patient Billing

The patient bill should reinforce the collection process while keeping the patient updated on the status of the account. Informing patients is particularly important for medical practices, since the practice may have to delay seeking payments from patients until the insurance companies have paid. To that end, some practices send the first bill to the patient 30 or more days after the service has been provided. By that time, the patient or guarantor may not recall the specifics of the visit or may not be familiar with complex insurance issues or payment rejections. In one example, a patient was billed for a service that was not covered because the patient did not meet the deductible. Because no explanation appeared on the bill, the patient called the practice for an explanation. The patient was annoyed, and the staff had to address the issue personally. A message on the bill about the filling of the insurance claim and the disposition of the insurance payment would have avoided the problem.

In most systems, the patient's demographic record contains a billing or account code, which is used to classify patients for billing. The code may be only a selection criteria for bill production. If so, the practice must tell the system which patients' codes should be selected for each billing run.

Other systems associate the code with a profile of billing standards. Standards include the actual bill design, selected aging messages, and minimum billing amounts. The standards may also include billing frequency and billing triggers. Billing frequency may be every 20 or 30 days, and billing triggers include insurance payments, patient payments, and new charges. This way, each time a financial transaction is posted to an account, a bill is sent to the patient. Many systems also allow the practice not to send a bill to a patient who has received a bill within a specified number of days.

Once bills are produced, some products will maintain an image of the bill, so that the practice's staff can call it up if they need to discuss the patient's account over the phone. The staff can see the information as the patient sees it. Note that some systems do not offer a display of the patient's account that in any way represents the bill that was sent to the patient. The lack of a bill-like listing complicates communication with the patient on billing matters.

A practice can avoid printing bills itself by shipping the electronic version of the bills to a service that will print out the bills, stuff the envelopes, and mail the bills. Such services are available from selected software vendors (e.g., +MEDIC) or from third-party billing organizations that use selected file dumps from any practice management system.

Insurance Billing

Many practices avoid billing insurance companies and hold the patient responsible for all insurance matters; others consider insurance billing a service to patients. Privately insured patients can find filling out forms time-consuming and confusing. Filing insurance forms for patients can ease the patients' paperwork and increase the chances of the practice getting paid directly—and quickly—by the insurance company.

For practices that do not accept assignment of payment or that require payment with service, insurance billing is not an issue. For other practices, insurance company or benefit plan tracking is a critical task. Billing for health maintenance organizations (HMOs) and preferred provider organizations (PPOs) is particularly troublesome. Each plan has a different approved fee and payment structure. There can be differences from one HMO or PPO to the next concerning what is an acceptable treatment. Insurance billing should be reinforced with company-specific collections, benefit calculation, and checking of reimbursements.

Insurance claims can be filed on paper or electronically. Many insurance companies require the industry standard HCFA 1500 claim form, which the practice prints on its computer and sends to the insurer. The computer must be programmed to insert various codes specific to each insurance company, such as provider IDs, location codes, and authorization information. Note that a variety of freestanding organizations require their own claim forms, which may differ dramatically from the HCFA 1500.

Electronic Claims

Electronic claims submission does enable practices to speed up the claims process, sometimes cutting two to four weeks off the insurance payment cycle. However, there are more than 750 different electronic claims structures among the established insurance companies. Many practice management systems handle only a few insurance companies that are particularly active in their target markets. The practice must choose software that can handle electronic claims for its most significant insurers.

Independent electronic claims clearinghouses can accept electronic claims for a variety of insurers at one time. The claims are sorted by insurer and passed on to the insurer. ENVOY/NEIC, CYDATA, and EQUIFAX are examples of claims clearinghouses.

More and more insurers also offer electronic EOBs. Electronic EOBs include the same details of payments from the insurance company as are found on paper EOBs. The original electronic claim is submitted with a practice claim number that is returned on the electronic EOB. The claim number is used to post the payment to the specific charge. Electronic posting of EOBs can save a great deal of time that is now dedicated to figuring out what the EOB is for and posting the payments and write-offs to each charge.

Systems handle the posting in a variety of ways. Some verify the payment against the expected payment, post automatic write-offs for participating plans, and promote the claim to the next insurer or the patient. Most vendors are still developing this capability, and many insurers do not offer electronic EOBs. The practice must choose software that can handle the requirement and that handles electronic EOBs for key local insurers.

COLLECTIONS

Every medical billing system includes an accounts receivable report that can be used for collection efforts. Unfortunately, the reports quickly become obsolete. As soon as a new patient is checked out or the daily checks are posted, the receivables report has to be redone.

The receivables report is merely a work list of accounts that meet the dollar value or aging selection criteria. Collection efforts must be documented on a separate piece of paper or in the patient's computer account record. For example, some practices set up a dummy "collections" provider in the appointment scheduling system. Commitments by patients or follow-ups with delinquent patients are scheduled on the appointment book for the nonexistent provider. This method does not allow for historically tracking either collection efforts or fulfillment of commitments.

Documenting collection efforts is especially important to practices that deal with a large number of insurers or must track multiple payment and collection issues. By logging appropriate due dates and payment commitments, the practice can keep up the pressure on problem accounts and refer serious problems to collection agencies sooner. On average, 20% of the bills sent to a collection agency are collected. The collection agency earns 35% of the money collected through its own efforts and 50% of fees gained through the courts. Obviously, practices have a significant incentive to work accounts as thoroughly as possible before transferring them to collection agencies.

Medical practices actually have two distinct collection problems: patients who do not pay and insurance companies. The failure of people to pay is not a problem unique to the medical industry. However, many patients are not aware of the various payment issues or the responsibility of the insurance company. The practice's staff must have information on insurance payments readily available to explain the status of the patient's obligation quickly and clearly.

A significant portion of payments for services to patients comes from insurance companies. However, each insurance company enforces a bewildering array of rules and claim-filing standards that challenges even the largest practices. To manage insurance companies, the practice needs to monitor the status of claims closely, verify insurance payments, and issue appropriate documentation to address any questions that have caused payments to be delayed. Note that many collection systems manage collections only from patients, when in fact the same tools are desperately needed to manage commitments and claims by insurance companies.

Attached to patient billing systems, collection management tools help the practice operate as a virtual collection agency. Indeed, some practices set up a separate phone line and post office box to give patients the impression that another organization is now collecting for the practice. In any case, a collection module provides a variety of tools to keep up with patients' bills and to follow up on payment commitments.

Initially, the operator selects a profile to assign accounts or transactions to collection status. The profile may include the age of the account, the dollar value of the amount owed, the service date, the days since last payment, or the number of bills sent. The selection process will move the appropriate accounts to collections using one of the following strategies:

1. **Tag the account or transaction and reclassify the amount due.** The account is coded as a collection account. The system may be set up to exclude the account from regular accounts by omitting accounts in that class. Usually the system will display a flashing message or some warning if someone tries to schedule an appointment or enter a charge for the account. In the patient account status, the system will display the collection amount next to the regular receivable amount. A patient could be in arrears for a portion of the account but current in another part of the account. Payments for collection amounts are posted directly to the patient's account and will be reflected in the management reports and practice analysis.

2. **Write off the amount transferred to collections and post the transactions to the collection system.** When the account or transaction is moved to collections, the amount is written off the patient's record through a special adjustment code. The amount disappears from the various receivables reports, so the patient account summary displays no outstanding amount. Payments are posted to a dummy account, or an adjustment is posted to the patient's account to write up the account so the payment can be posted. If posted to a dummy account, the collected funds will not be reflected in procedure-based analysis. More important, the patient's balance of zero obscures the collection issues at the level of the patient. The patient's outstanding charges may not be easily detected from appointment scheduling or other patient service screens.

Once an account is in collections, the system should provide a selection of collector tools. Typically, the user can select an account from a work list of all of the accounts assigned to the collector or from a list of pending-action items based on a tickler date. Once an account is selected, the typical software displays a summary of the account information, including the aged balance, special notes, and any outstanding commitments. After reviewing the account, the collector may contact the patient. Some systems even support automatic dialing of the selected phone number over a modem.

For the collections staff to work with the responsible party over the phone, the collection screen should allow quick access to the patient ledger, transaction details, and other system information. The collector should be able to send a statement, print a letter, file a claim, and note the contact—all from the same screen. Similarly, the collector should be able to record the results of the effort, including getting a payment commitment, posting a credit card payment, or establishing a payment plan.

The collection system should support all the necessary follow-up tasks, including managing a payment plan and placing a dated commitment on the collector work list. The commitment would be displayed for the collector on the due date.

RECEIPTS

Receipts posting varies according to the open item strategy of the software. (For a more detailed explanation of open item strategies, see "Open Item Accounting" earlier in this chapter.) In some systems, the operator simply enters the amount of the check or adjustment and the charges are paid off on an FIFO, proportional, or selected basis.

Billing has a direct impact on the posting of receipts. Systems that support insurance company-specific fee schedules allow for an insurer-specific fee schedule, expected approved (or usual and customary) amount, and payment amount. The specific fee schedules are used to handle negotiated reduced-fee arrangements as well as standard participating provider arrangements.

For reduced-fee arrangements, the practice should enter the negotiated fee schedule as the billing amount. Bills will be sent out at the reduced fee, and the receivables will reflect the reduced fee. For standard participating provider arrangements the standard fee would be billed, because the usual and customary fee is not necessarily known. Indeed, the usual and customary fee can change at any time.

Company-specific amounts will be used to prompt the user when insurance checks are being posted, and the user can verify that the insurance company paid the right amount. If the insurance company paid the wrong amount, then the practice will submit an inquiry to get the right amount.

When the charge is entered, some software packages will automatically calculate the expected payment from the insurance company as well as the projected write-off. The calculated amounts can be accepted, or the EOB amount can be entered. The write-off will be assigned a code for that particular insurance company. The write-off code allows management reports to compile summary realization and write-off information correctly. As an option, the user can update the expected charge and payment directly from the payment posting screen.

Patient payments can be posted to a particular charge or date of service. If the patient has not specified how to apply the payment, the practice could apply the payment to old charges or allow for an unapplied payment that may be posted to charges later. There are some practical challenges to posting patient payments. In theory, only charges that are the patient's responsibility would be paid by a patient payment. Indeed, some systems track patient and insurance obligations separately. A patient could have a credit in the patient balance, while insurance receivables remain. However, a patient may send a check that represents an insurance payment.

These issues pose significant challenges to billing. However, maintaining accurate open item receivables is the only way to ensure that the management report summaries are based on an accurate distribution of receipts. The open item distribution information is the key to monitoring contracts, realization, and performance.

Note that insurance check handling varies widely. In some cases, each patient's account is posted separately. Separate posting usually results in a deposit ticket that lists each application of a check but not a total for a check. The deposit report would appear as if many checks had been entered, when in fact an single check for an EOB had been applied to many patients.

Regardless of the posting method, proper posting of insurance checks is the key to using the computer—both to manage fee realization and to monitor the practice's insurance company relationships.

PRACTICE PERFORMANCE MEASURES

To deal with rapidly changing business and management issues, a medical practice must apply more sophisticated business management techniques. Unfortunately, to fill this need many practice management systems can generate data but little information. Being able to identify basic trends and business measures from all that data can do a great deal to help the practice manage and monitor its performance. Many practice management products include multiple transaction reports but few management reports. Management reports need to include realization statistics and trend analysis of revenues, payments, and billings, and they should be available for individual locations in a multiple-office practice, for individual providers, and for practices as a whole.

Note that many systems include summary reports that can be compiled into meaningful performance monitoring tools. For example, software to perform trend analysis over time is not included with many systems, but an appropriate spreadsheet maintained from period reports can provide a meaningful performance tracking tool.

Some useful performance measures include:

- Receivables days outstanding
- Comparing charges to payments and adjustments on a daily and a monthly basis
- Reports—by provider, office, and insurer—of the total charges and resulting payments

EVOLVING PERFORMANCE MEASURES

One of the critical junctures to consider in the selection of a computer system is the reporting issues that the practice will face in the future:

- **Outcome measurement** Outcome measurement monitors the patient condition, patient satisfaction, and clinical results of the services, as well as the protocols used to treat the patient. Outcomes may be based on specific diagnostic testing as well as on survival rates. In order to measure outcomes, the system must combine service and treatment information with the patient status at a future time.
- **Quality assurance** Quality assurance is based on measuring various treatment and service factors against a standard or goal. A wide variety of quality assurance factors are possible; they could cover everything from the time a patient waits in the office to see a provider to determining if patient wellness standards (e.g., well baby visits) are being completed. Quality assurance reporting requires reporting on the clinical status and treatment status of patients compared to the quality measurement.
- **Utilization management and measurement** Utilization management and measurement require the availability of treatment protocols and/or standards that can be compared to the actual experience of the practice. Utilization management and measurement require tracking of in-house services as well as hospital, lab, and other providers.

To produce reports of value, the system must collect the information for the report as a natural by-product of the patient service process. The information needed for the reports must be entered in the system as the patient is served or treated, and not after the fact. If the practice collects this information on a historical basis, the data will be subject to interpretation, errors, and/or missing information. For example, some practices must compile information on a manual report for an outcome measurement service. The information is derived from patient diagnostic and service information for an eight-to-ten month period.

These reporting options will require some of the advanced features mentioned elsewhere in this book (e.g., treatment plans and office routing). The capabilities must be supported by a fully functional and comprehensive electronic medical record.

CHAPTER 5 • MANAGED CARE

CONTENTS

5 MANAGED CARE

A complete set of information is needed to ensure that a medical practice can meet the recordkeeping and administrative requirements of managed care cost-effectively. Under the fee-for-service model, which until recently was widely prevalent, a straightforward relationship exists among the patient schedule, the charge, and the medical record (see Figure 4). A practice was free to manage patient information as it saw fit.

Unfortunately, few, if any, practices maintained all the information and all of the cross-references between key areas of patient information. How practices kept and used information was an internal issue. Practices that did maintain all of the necessary administrative information resorted to additional staff and cumbersome procedures. For example, pediatricians used a face sheet to record immunizations that were also in the medical record for the day of service as well as in the patient billing record. The medical record and face sheet were recorded separately by hand.

MANAGED CARE SOFTWARE NEEDS

Under managed care, an increasing number of parties seek information from the medical practice's records. Insurers want practices to maintain certain information about treatments, and hospitals and insurance companies want the practice to enter information into their computer systems. Practices that are managing other aspects of a patient's health want more

Figure 4: Standard Internal Relationships

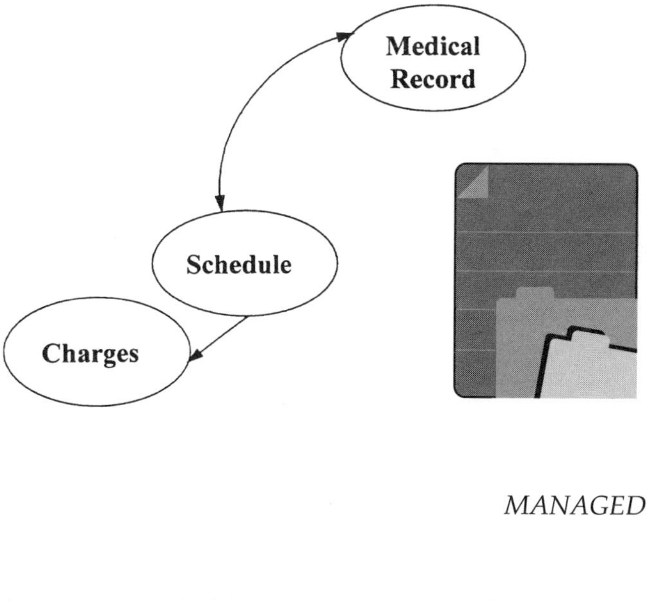

Medical Record

Schedule

Charges

Figure 5: Managed Care—Internal Relationships

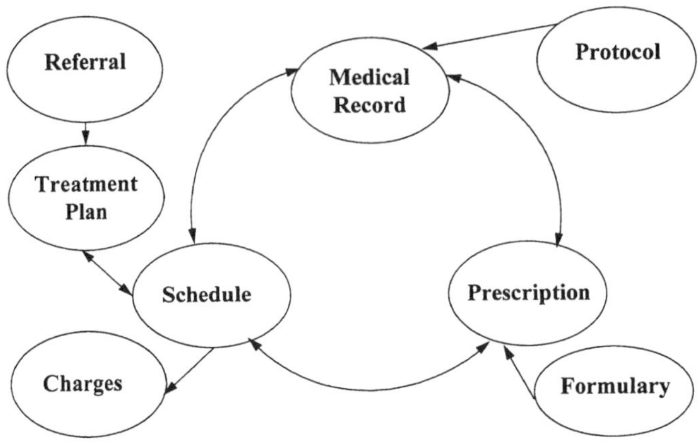

information from primary care providers (PCPs) in order to control costs and improve patient services. Governing all of these efforts are more and more rules for practitioners to follow and enforce while treating patients.

Managed care programs may define drug formulations, treatment protocols, and patient service standards. Other initiatives seek to establish cooperative relationships among providers and insurers to manage chronic illness and costly diseases. To manage these data items internally requires a more complex structure than was previously used. See Figure 5, which illustrates how the medical record information is now related to additional controls and data items. The additional information is used to access the various terms and conditions of each plan as well as to manage information about each patient. The treatment plan defines what services can appropriately be scheduled for the patient. The medical record then documents those services to the patient. Failure to maintain the standards of each insurer could result in a utilization problem or in treating a patient without first completing the authorization process.

More important, under managed care the practice has a great need to relate the medical record to the treatment protocol and the patient schedule. Practices that try to manage these tasks manually spend more staff time tracking additional paper and make less money while they're doing it. For example, some practices use special face sheets or intake forms to store insurer-specific information in the patient's record. Those practices would have to physically retrieve and review every relevant patient file to compile statistical abstracts or prove compliance.

Because each managed care plan has different rules and different participating providers, managing patients' needs within a plan becomes an administrative challenge. For example, a primary care practice may be requested to gather information on whether its patients' children regularly use seat belts, or a specialist may be required to obtain preapproval for services not on the referral authorization. Regardless of the basic operational and patient management issues, practices still must fulfill managed care commitments—and must do so economically. To avoid an unbearable administrative cost, practices must seek software that supports compliance with managed care plans.

In one sense, providers merely need to focus on the needs of additional customers of the practice. These customers might be insurers, employers who manage their own health plans, a hospital-based plan through a physician–hospital organization, or a plan administered by an independent provider association. The practice must have a computer system that lets it operate within the specific parameters of each plan.

As a practical matter, practices will not be able to track every rule and every provider in every plan in their area. They should be able to track the plans that are most important, however, and on a cost-effective basis. Most practices under the fee-for-service environment have only a handful of plans that account for much of their activity. Under managed care, the number of active plans will be limited to those that produce the most patients. This is similar to a fee-for-service environment in which Blue Shield, Medicare, and a few commercial plans dominate the claim activity for many practices.

MANAGED CARE RELATIONSHIPS

Before undertaking any evaluation or selection effort, the practice must recognize the pervasive and dramatic effect that the evolving managed care environment has on the practice and the general healthcare marketplace.

Managed care is a term used to describe a number of changes that have taken place in the healthcare environment over the past few years. In general, managed care seeks to fit all providers (e.g., physicians, hospitals, laboratories) into a more "rational" or organized healthcare delivery model. This rather basic objective is complicated by the fact that so many of the constituencies involved have differing views of what a rational healthcare delivery model should look like. A variety of ideas has been proposed, including a single insurance entity to replace more than 1,500 healthcare insurers; regional healthcare delivery models to coordinate care among literally thousands of providers in a geographic area; cooperative integrated delivery systems that enable thousands of providers to work together; and a host of other entities, acronyms, and logos. Whether any one of these strategies will become the standard in a particular area is not necessarily important. The bottom line is that more managed care models will appear, along with new approaches to improve patient care and control costs. Many practices will be dealing with a variety of cooperative working relationships as well as some variation of the fee-for-service model.

Which, if any, of these models becomes significant will depend on whether any of them can ultimately save money for those businesses, insurers, government agencies, and patients who pay the bills. For the time being, practices must accommodate a number of operational methodologies and standards to work with a variety of healthcare plans.

Before reviewing specific managed care issues, practices must consider that most of the medical practice software on the market today was written originally to manage the fee-for-service environment. To meet managed care needs, many vendors are hooking into the standard fee-for-service system. When choosing software, a medical practice should be certain that the product chosen maintains enough checkpoints to keep data on the managed care system "in sync" with data on the fee-for-service system. For example, a patient treatment plan on the medical records product must be capable of verifying appointments scheduled on the practice management system. When a patient is being scheduled for an appointment, the office staff should be able to check the need for a referral authorization and attach the appointment to the referral authorization information.

When evaluating systems for managed care issues, the practice must be certain that the system actually addresses all the issues discussed in the following sections.

PATIENT PANEL MANAGEMENT

Patient panels are lists of patients covered under a particular plan. Under fee-for-service plans, providers who did not participate in an insurance company's plan looked to the patient for payment; whether the payment came from a patient, a guarantor, or an insurance company was not particularly important. Under managed care plans, however, the patient panel represents those patients who have chosen or been assigned to the practice.

A provider uses a patient panel to perform the following tasks.

- **Verify that patients are covered under the capitation payment.** The patient panel can be used to verify the capitation payment or per-patient charge for each patient. Without the patient panel, the provider cannot verify the amount or be certain the patient is covered. Payments for each patient may be based on sex, age, occupation code, and/or location. The complete patient panel should be kept in the system for primary care providers.

  Some systems keep all eligible patients in the patient master files. Other products maintain separate files for eligible patients and active patients. If a newly active patient is not found in the patient file, the basic patient information in the eligibility file can be copied to set up a new patient record. Most practices check paper lists to verify patient eligibility and plan terms.
- **Select patients for wellness services.** Under some managed care contracts, primary care providers manage wellness services for appropriate patients in the panel. For example, a provider may commit to providing an annual physical examination to patients of a certain age. The system should be able to identify patients according to a certain profile. A letter or automatic tickler file record could be generated for

each patient who meets the selection criteria. The practice could select all males over age 55 and send them an informational letter on prostate issues, for example.

- **Serve patients.** Staff can project a more responsive image by managing persons on the patient panel who have yet to visit the practice. The practice could send a letter of introduction and welcome to patients who are new to the practice. Being able to select a patient from the eligibility file quickly will ease the initial intake of patient information.

Verifying the payment against the patient panel is relatively easy for PCPs, since a single provider may manage only a few thousand patients. However, specialists may receive a payment that covers services for tens of thousands of patients, yet many of those capitated patients will never be seen by the specialist.

The practice also may wish to determine why patients leave the panel. This information could be gathered through a statistical survey or when patients call for release of records to a new provider. In this way, the practice could identify problem areas in its own operation as well as convey any insurance company issues to the appropriate contacts.

SERVICE PANELS

Under the fee-for-service model, providers generally are free to provide services they deem appropriate and necessary. Under managed care plans, however, the practice may be limited to certain procedures or groups of procedures on the basis of a certification process (plans accept providers based on capabilities and other factors), the need to provide certain services in a geographic area of the plan, and/or cost. For example, one managed care plan required all lab work to be routed to a particular lab, since that lab could complete tests at less cost than other outside labs or office labs.

Each practice may also be limited to certain procedures on the basis of the managed care contract. For example, perhaps only a certain set of procedures is covered under a capitated plan, but the practice may also provide services that can be billed to the plan separately. Or a practice may be forbidden to provide specific services. If the practice provides a service that is not covered under the agreement, the plan or referring provider may refuse payment. The practice could then incur the cost of services but not receive compensation from the plan.

A service could be covered, billed separately, or excluded from the plan completely. These three attributes could differ by procedure code for each plan. Because most systems can assign only a charge value to a procedure, an employee would not be prevented from posting a charge that has not been authorized or excluded for the practice. Unfortunately, such information cannot be handled through a fee schedule, since it would be difficult to determine which procedures are included and which are completely excluded.

REFERRALS

Primary care providers and specialists alike may refer a patient to another provider for a variety of reasons. Under fee-for-service systems, a provider may recommend that a patient see another provider for further examination, lab tests, radiology studies, or a consultation. In almost all fee-for-service cases, it is up to the patient to select and contact that second provider. In some cases, the patient may not seek the referred services, and the primary care provider may not find out that the patient has failed to seek additional help until the primary care provider checks up on the patient. This may delay treatment.

Under managed care, the referring provider directs the patient to a specific provider. Unfortunately, this is not as simple as it sounds, because each plan is different. Each provider may offer a different set of services for each plan. For example, a doctor may be able to perform his or her own lab tests under one managed care plan, but the doctor must refer all lab tests to a particular lab under a second managed care plan. A third managed care plan might allow that same lab to perform certain lab tests but require a series of tests to be routed to yet another lab. Similar arrangements are required for radiology and other specialties.

Referral Providers

All managed care providers must manage and deal with a larger network of providers. Once a doctor has determined that a patient needs to be referred to another provider, he or she must determine the appropriate party on the basis of the provider's participation in the appropriate plan,

Figure 6: Managed Care—PCP View

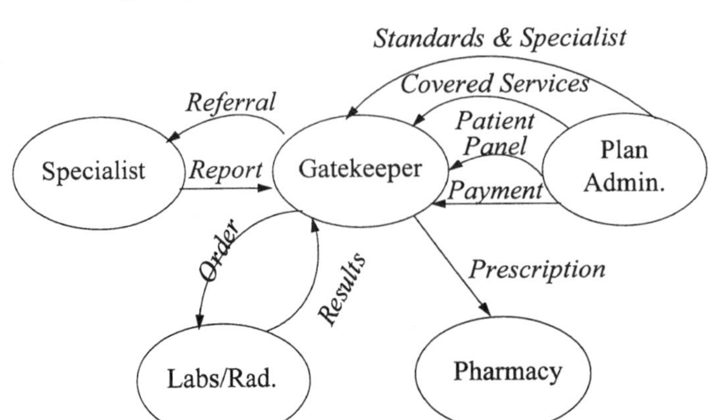

Figure 7: Managed Care—Specialist View

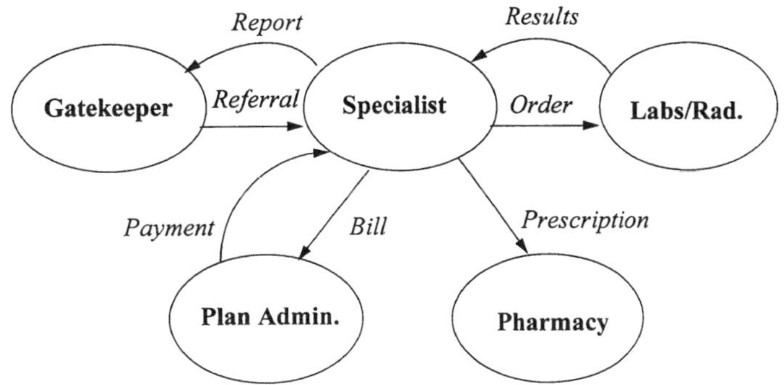

the patient's preferences (such as location), and whether the provider is authorized to provide the needed services. Making such a selection takes time.

Practice management systems can speed the selection of providers by accommodating referring-provider profiles. A set of services or practice areas may be associated with a provider for each plan. The provider may have a different relationship with each plan. In addition to credentialing (a process by which a plan reviews an applicant's credentials to determine whether to admit him or her as an accepted provider for a set of services), some plans may limit the number of providers who can offer certain services. The provider profile is used to select an appropriate provider for outpatient services.

Referral Authorizations

In the managed care environment, the PCP monitors services provided to a patient as well as authorizing the level of care or services provided by other providers. The referral authorization acts as a "service authorization" from the provider to the specialist, lab, or other party. The entire process from the perspective of the PCP perspective can be found in Figure 6. Figure 7 illustrates the referral authorization process from the specialist's perspective.

Referral authorizations are addressed to a particular provider. Indeed, the provider may not be compensated for services from the plan if the appropriate referral authorization is not generated and passed onto the plan's third-party administrator. Depending on the plan, the provider who issues the referral authorization may specify limitations. In some cases, referral authorizations have no limits, but in many cases, limits are imposed on the number of visits and the dates when the visits may occur. Some plans limit the dollar value of the referral authorization, the types of procedures that may be performed, or both. In the most specific cases, the provider authorizes specific procedure codes. For example, a referral authorization may specify that up to $200 may be provided for up to five office visits.

From a practice management standpoint, the referral authorization represents "booked" services. The practice can track the value of future services to measure performance and patient services. The referral authorization also limits treatment, however, and requires a higher level of administrative effort to direct patients to the correct provider. Practices must maintain all of the various records related to managed care.

Ideally, the referral authorization should be connected to the appointment scheduler, charges, and the patient ledger. Thereby, the practice can track the various activities that are associated with each referral authorization.

RISK MANAGEMENT

Providers may have to assume the risk of loss through capitation. Under capitation, a managed care plan allots a practice a certain sum of money each month for each covered patient. The allowed fee per patient may vary by age, sex, and plan. In some cases, capitation payments even vary by location. Indeed, the risk assumed by the practice may vary by a number of factors, including the covered services.

Additionally, there are several hybrid payment forms, such as the following:

- **Patient visit or "threshold" payments** The practice receives a certain amount of money for each patient visit. If the time needed to see the patient is only a few minutes, the practice has made money; but if the patient requires a battery of tests, the practice may lose money on that particular patient.
- **Diagnostic group payments** The practice is paid a certain amount of money on the basis of the diagnosis. If the practice solves the problem with less effort and fewer services than the insurance company has projected, the practice makes money. If the practice has to work with the patient for an extended treatment period, the practice may lose money on that particular patient.

All forms of risk assumption may be covered by a stop-loss provision, by which the provider can bill the plan for a reduced fee for services beyond a certain level. For example, a provider may have to provide only the first $10,000 of services to a patient. Charges beyond the stop-loss may be paid by the insurance company on a reduced-fee basis. Although the exact calculation varies by insurer, the practice management system chosen should be able to identify those accounts that could cause problems.

Managing risk is a challenge for any practice management system. In general, most systems attempt to track capitation performance and risk through the familiar fee-for-service model. The patient accounting for managed care can result in any number of problems, depending on the strategy used for charge and payment posting.

Posting Capitated Charges

Figure 8, which illustrates the basic capitation posting strategies used by most vendors, shows the effect of standard payment charge posting, zero charge with a co-payment (co-pay) charge, and posting capitated charges at standard and writing off the difference. The effect on patient ledgers, statements, management reports, and realization can be clarified as follows.

If the co-pay is entered as a separate charge and the actual procedure is entered as a zero, the patient statements are correct but most management reports will count the procedure as a zero charge. A detailed procedure analysis report will understate realization for the procedure, since no charge or revenue will be credited to the procedure.

If the charge is set to the co-pay, most systems will use the co-pay as the value of the service. Therefore, the charges will be understated and realization will not include the capitated payment or the full value of the services.

Posting the charge at standard and writing off the difference between the co-pay and the charge will complicate patients' statements. The work needed to manage this process is quite demanding and is practical only if the system is designed to manage capitated charges in this manner.

Capitated check posting poses another challenge. Figure 9 illustrates posting capitated checks. The effect on realization is indicated as "no effect," "understated," or "overstated."

Frequently, the capitation check from the plan administrator is not entered into the practice management system. Because the check is not in the system, realization reports will not include the revenue at any level. This results in misleading realization reports. Audit trails will be less than clear, because the receipt register from the practice management system will not match the actual deposits.

Posting the payment to a dummy account will keep the receipts in balance but may misstate charges. If charges are misstated, then realization reports will be incorrect.

Posting the payment to patient accounts like an insurance explanation of benefits (EOB) will maintain the integrity of the practice management system, but it could be labor-intensive. The operator must first calculate the realization and then go back into a detailed posting to each account with activity.

Systems that have been designed to handle capitation checks use a separate insurance account. This approach maintains the integrity of the system and allows the practice to manage the relationship with the insurance company.

When selecting a medical software system, practices should be sure to fully consider the accounting and reporting implications of posting capitated charges and checks.

Figure 8: Capitated Plan Charge Posting

	Units	FFS	Zero Charge	Set to Co-pay	Post at Standard Charge	Post at Standard Write Off	Post at Standard Net
OV	1	60	0	10	60	50	10
Lab Test	1	25	0	0	25	25	0
Co-pay	1	N/A	10	N/A	N/A	N/A	N/A
Patient Ledger		✔	–	–		✔	
Patient Statements		✔	✔	✔		?	
Management Reports		✔	–	–		✔	
Realization		✔	–	?		✔	

Figure 9: Capitated Plan Payment Posting

Option	*Receipts*	*Charges*	*Realization*
Outside System	U	O/U	U
Dummy Account	=	O/=	U/=
Patient Accounts	=	=	=
Insurance Account	=	=	=

U: understated; O: overstated; =: no effect

CLAIMS ADJUDICATION

Sometimes providers must pass patients on to other providers for services they have contracted for but cannot provide. The referring providers set up their own relationship with the outside providers and pay the patients' bills directly from the funds they receive from the plan. Third-party payment administrators that are evolving to act solely to engage the services of outside providers will become an important requirement for these groups.

As yet, many of these groups lack the volume of referrals or covered lives to justify a complete third-party administration (TPA) system. TPA systems include many of the features needed to function as an insurance company: They track eligible patients, providers, and service authorizations, and they can accept provider billing information, verify payment rates, and issue checks to providers. A complete set of management reports would cover payables management as well as realization and utilization.

TPA systems include modules to track provider credentialing and plan administration. Such systems start at $100,000. Even though a complete

TPA system may not be needed, some practices need to be able handle payments to outside providers efficiently and measure future outstanding authorizations. Even if an outside TPA system is in use, the treatment status information remains a significant part of the patient record as well as a trigger for payment.

A basic claims adjudication process that manages the payment process and produces comprehensive risk and payables information would be useful for a variety of management service organization (MSO)–type entities. Such a module would produce the check, manage cash flow, and maintain the appropriate audit trails for the referral authorization, completion of services, and compensation of outside providers.

QUALITY ASSURANCE

Depending on its contract with the managed care plan, the practice may be responsible for providing a certain level of service to patients. In addition to allowed services, primary care providers may be responsible for defined preventive care programs. For example, the provider may have to see children according to a specified standard in the first year of life.

Quality assurance measures encompass everything from the time a patient first contacts the practice until the patient changes providers, even if the provider never sees the patient. The key to measuring quality assurance is to have a flexible report writer that accumulates summary information and easily selects exceptions.

Some systems include a selection and report feature that allows the practice to select patients based on values in their demographic or charge records. For example, the practice could search for all patients who have a particular diagnosis and have been treated during a certain span of time. These patient lists could be used to evaluate some care standards.

Other information from the appointment scheduling system could be used to monitor patient flow, or the time that elapses between a patient's telephone call and the scheduling of an appointment. A wide variety of service and clinical metrics can be used to measure quality. As long as the system can capture and retain the information and a flexible report writer can search it, the practice will be able to look at quality measures at the top level (e.g., patients with a particular condition who have not been seen in a certain number of months) and use the system to review quality from other angles (e.g., patients with the condition who *were* seen or potential risk groups). These tools will generate performance measures for the practice and help the practice pursue patient wellness effectively.

CHAPTER 6 • MEDICAL RECORDS

CONTENTS

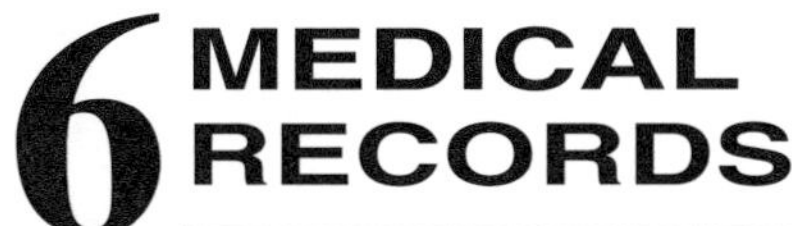

6 MEDICAL RECORDS

Use of computerized patient charts across the healthcare industry is the ultimate goal of a number of organizations. For example, insurers want providers to maintain adequate, accessible records to allow insurance companies and medical practices to manage compliance easily. In fact, some insurers offer malpractice insurance discounts to practices that use electronic medical records. Advocates of integrated delivery systems foresee the exchange of electronic medical charts among providers.

While medical practices show a high level of interest in using electronic medical records, the reality is that few practices are in a position to implement an electronic system successfully. Many medical record initiatives have failed to meet the real needs of physicians and add value to the practice. This is often due to the staff's lack of clear objectives and failure to understand the system.

THE ADVANTAGES OF ELECTRONIC MEDICAL RECORDS

Medical records document the important and costly exchange between patient and doctor. If a practice can identify enough uses of patient information, and these needs are the driving force behind a medical record effort, then the practice may be able to use electronic medical records effectively.

Examples of uses include the following:

1. **Providers can monitor patient trends and wellness.** The medical data gathered over time can then be analyzed to help patients as well as to monitor trends in the patient population. Providers could define a profile, based on various demographic, treatment, and practice-defined information, of patients who the provider wishes to contact. For example, patients who have a condition that requires continual medication but who have not renewed their prescription in a year could be contacted. The system could select patients according to the profile and send a letter, place a message in their records, or put their names on an action list.
2. **Patients who received a drug, a medical device, or treatment that was later found to create a long-term problem can be easily identified.** If the various treatments and prescriptions were entered

into the system, for example, a search could be initiated to identify patients with a certain condition who have been prescribed a particular drug. The list could be used to contact the patients.

3. **Practices can verify that adequate documentation is captured according to their treatment procedures and protocols.** If a practice uses standardized flow sheets or patient chart forms, then a certain level of standardization can be established over the medical records. If those standard clinical forms were in a computer system, the computer could identify medical records that have not been filled out or even initiated. For example, if a patient's vital signs have not been taken for a physical, this fact would show up on a list of incomplete medical records. Such a list could not be produced in a cost-effective way using manual records. Also, identify those medical records that have not been filled out or even initiated. For example, if a patient's vital signs have not been taken for a physical, this would show up on a list of imcomplete medical records. The appropriate records could then be completed. Thereby, the practice could have a higher degree of confidence in committing to various outside standards or responding to surveys for insurers and employers. Compliance with recording standards could be determined easily, and providers could be evaluated on the accuracy and completeness of their records.
4. **Medical records can be accessed from the provider's home and from other service locations.** During off hours, providers must rely on memory or on the recollections of patients. If electronic medical records are available, the provider can call into the office system and review a patient's treatment history or issues from home. The electronic medical record would be easily referenced because the information would be organized by the medical record system, and the electronic medical record would be easy to read. The provider could also record the disposition of the problem and leave an action item for the next business day.
5. **As the average practice increases in size, automated medical records increase staff flexibility.** Computer records allow a larger practice to provide a consistent level of service. Having a standardized record establishes the patient's information as an asset of the practice that can be used to bond the practice to the patient and not just the patient to the provider. Some medical record systems include a single screen abstract of key information, from which the provider can quickly examine continuing problems, current prescriptions, and other information for the patient. If necessary, the provider can dig down into more detailed information or the patient's history. By standardizing the records, physicians and clinical staff will be able to access information easily because all of the medical records follow a standard methodology. When a covering doctor is reviewing the records of another doctor's patient, no adjustments will need to be made for different recordkeeping methods or handwriting differences. Thereby a number of different providers will be able to work with one patient quickly and effectively.

6. **Aggregate reports can be easily produced.** To serve patients and employers better, a practice can aggregate data on incidents and conditions in order to identify trends and monitor patient wellness. Such statistical analysis might include utilization measures to identify effective treatment protocols and providers as well as to evaluate the effectiveness of the practice as a whole. Aggregate reports also measure compliance with managed care requirements and standards; for example, the practice could document the results of its efforts to get men over age 40 to participate in physical wellness programs.
   These analyses and documents could be used to address various issues proactively as well as challenge the information and/or analyses of various outside parties who may be reviewing practice performance. For example, a managed care organization may challenge a practice on utilization. It will be to the advantage of the managed care organization to consider various clinically significant issues with the patient population in a computer-generated analysis.

THE CHALLENGES OF COMPUTERIZED MEDICAL RECORDS

The benefits of automated medical records can clearly be made to outweigh the costs of acquiring and recording the information. Access to the system is required from each service delivery point in the practice's office as well as from remote locations. Hospital-based providers may need access to information kept in the office system, and providers may want to verify treatment plans and drugs from home when they are on call. Computerized recordkeeping can dramatically decrease the time needed to find medical records and dramatically increase the accessibility of information. Several insurance companies also offer discounts for practices that use computerized medical records.

Larger organizations in particular can benefit from the variety of information and management tools to be derived from medical records. Medical records play a central role in justifying treatment, as well as meeting the needs of the many users who want access to treatment information on an aggregate basis. Using computers to survey the information in the medical records will help management measure provider performance, assess the overall health of covered groups, and identify areas in which to focus resources. A variety of outside sources also have a legitimate need to access specific information or review summary information.

The use of computerized medical records is a major challenge because of several issues, including the following:

1. **Computerized medical records are costly to acquire and to implement.** Deploying medical records electronically in a practice requires a much more extensive and robust technology infrastructure. Workstations must be placed throughout the installation, and communica-

tions must be established to exchange information with other providers and remote locations. Additional investments in hardware are needed to allow for continued operations and to protect against the loss of data. However, the hidden costs are even more dramatic. Designing and establishing a common medical record scheme for a practice will require physician time. A provider committee must establish the clinical information that is needed as well as the compliance information for reporting to plan administrators or meeting National Center for Quality Assurance requirements. The medical record may need to include information that will support outcome measurement and performance tracking.

2. **Computerized medical records will require a dramatic change in the way physicians interact with patients.** Physicians who are taught to think independently may find it difficult to adhere to a standard methodology of investigating patients' problems. Indeed, some physicians feel that too much structure will prevent them from using their knowledge in the most efficient, effective manner. Many physicians have developed their own ways of treating patients, and they will question the benefits of standardization.
3. **Physicians may not have the time or inclination to enter treatment information into a system.** Few providers want to serve a patient over a terminal screen. The patient may be intimidated, and the data entry and technical issues may draw attention away from patient service issues. Entering the data later places an additional time burden on the physician. In order to capture the medical record as a natural by-product of the patient service process, the computer entry device must be unobtrusive and easy for the physician to use.
4. **A substantial body of patient information must be in the system for it to be an effective tool.** As long as the patient's history remains in the paper clinical record, providers would have to consult both paper and electronic records, which may be more cumbersome than continuing to use paper records. Depending on the practice and patient population, paper may be eliminated in a few months or it could take years.

Ironically, many practices already use some form of electronic medical records but rely primarily on paper for access to information for providers and others. WordPerfect, Word, and other word processing software packages are the most commonly used "electronic" medical record tools. The typical medical practice transcribes the patient record from an audio tape, a message service, or even the handwritten notes of the provider. Medical records are entered into a word processing system as a single file for all transcription or as a continuous medical record file for each patient. Some practices even put all transcription for a day for all patients in a single file.

When a single file is used for all transcription, all of the transcription information for a particular provider or for all the providers is entered into a single word processing file. Each patient's portion is tagged with the patient's name and pertinent identifying information. The document for each patient is printed and then placed in the clinical file.

When a continuous medical record file is used for each patient, a separate word processing file is maintained for each user, and the latest information is entered at the beginning or end of the file. The relevant page is printed and placed in the clinical record.

Medical records kept through simple word processing systems can be as expensive to maintain as electronic medical records but produce far fewer benefits. The primary expense of maintaining either record is the time required to enter the treatment information into either system. However, the word processing system does not maintain a link with the underlying service records in the medical management system; nor does it structure the information to make the record easy to locate. Each provider may organize his or her dictated record in a different way, or one provider may organize information in a different way even among patients who received the same treatment. The practice management system will not necessarily lead the user to the specific word processing file or even the right place in a large medical record file. Because there are no controls over word processing file changes, it would be easy for anyone who can access the file to change or delete information. In the final analysis, the provider will need to see the printed record, since that record should be correct.

Because of such disadvantages to using word processing systems for medical records, many medical practices will derive greater benefit from investing in transcriptionists if they use a medical records product to protect and structure the clinical information. Note that some medical records products use standard word processors to enter medical records but download the word processing information into a medical record structure, thereby allowing the flexibility of a word processing package and the protection and patient management features of a medical records product.

Electronic medical records are especially useful for increasing efficiency among providers and staff. The electronic medical record allows the practice itself to define and then use a standard recording methodology. Once that methodology is defined, all the providers—including those who share patients, treatment responsibilities, or cross-coverage—will be dealing with fewer variations in recordkeeping and accessing of medical record information. This may save providers time and allow patients to be treated on the basis of more reliable information than their own recollections.

ENTRY STRATEGIES

Electronic medical records are entered into a medical record infrastructure through any one of several modes.

Keyboard

Historically, transcriptionists have typed medical records. Medical transcriptionists have knowledge of medical terminology and can interpret the speech or writing of the provider. For example, a provider may use a kind of shorthand to describe an evaluation as "normal," and the transcriptionist will expand the normal evaluation into appropriate language for the particular factor.

More and more providers are trying to keep medical records themselves, typically as a personal medical record for the provider. Keyboarding medical records is time-consuming and may distract patients if providers record information at the time of service. Recording information after serving the patient may take valuable time that could be used serving other patients.

Keyboarding can be speeded up through the use of a variety of entry tools. Standard responses can be called up in a few keystrokes. For example, the practice could use special "macros" for specific responses to a condition. A template file for a standard report format could easily be copied and filled in.

Scanning

Scanning allows the image of a previously recorded or newly documented medical record to be stored in the computer. Many of these documents can be interpreted by the computer only if the document was originally written to be scanned at a later date, yet few medical records are designed for later scanning. If they are so designed, the image of the document is stored according to user instructions or a special tag placed on the document—for example, the patient's number typed in the upper left-hand corner of the medical record.

Users can call up the document at a later date according to the special tag. However, the computer will not be able to search the text of the image for relevant information or to abstract information about a patient or a class of patients.

"Pen" Writing

Pen entry devices interpret the writing of the provider as he or she writes on a computer tablet. The computer tablet looks like a thick clipboard and weighs a few pounds. The user taps the pen on the line or field he or she wishes to enter and proceeds to write the information. As the user prints, the computer interprets the printed characters and displays a letter for each letter entered.

Pen writing systems can be used as a patient record for the provider alone or saved for later transmission to a central system, or they can interact directly with the central system through a direct connection or radio waves.

Voice

Voice systems convert the spoken word to written text. However, voice systems do not interpret the intent of the speaker or allow interpretations of the speaker to produce an effective medical record. For example, if a provider says "Normal," the voice system will recognize the word *normal* rather than the shorthand meaning a medical transcriptionist or a specially written macro would understand.

Many transcriptionists also correct grammar, fine-tune syntax, and clean up the flow of a report as they transcribe. Although expanding the word *normal* into a standard wording for the medical record is not difficult, modifying the *normal* to fit the situation and correcting the grammar are not as easy or straightforward.

CAPABILITIES OF ELECTRONIC MEDICAL RECORDS

Many medical records systems include a variety of standard information sets for common record items. Standard diagnoses, continuing problems, notes, prescriptions, and even patients' histories are provided with a number of systems. Some systems keep drug, dosage, instructions, and refill information for prescriptions. Systems are also available that will retain the various results from lab tests. In addition to standard information, the practice can add relevant information into medical record infrastructures that have been customized for the practice. Figure 10 illustrates some typical relationships. Medical record infrastructures include free-form, defined-forms, knowledge-base, and language-modeling formats.

Free-Form Format

The word processing medical record, which is an example of a free-form medical record, could range from a formal medical record to a referring physician letter. Because of the limitations of word processing systems, the exact file being sought may not be easy to find. Transcriptionists must follow a strict format and document summary standards to ensure that it will be easy to locate a file for a particular patient.

Other systems allow the provider to enter free-form text into a medical record format that is similar to a SOAP note. SOAP notes divide encounter information into Subjective, Objective, Analysis, and Plan sections. The Subjective portion includes the provider's observations and the patient's description of the problem, while the Objective section may include vital statistics, measurements, and lab tests. The Analysis portion documents the provider's review of the information and diagnostic conclusion. The Plan section may prescribe a drug or lay out an extended treatment plan.

Free-form medical records are easy to use, and they do not require dramatic changes in operations because they do not impose standards. Free-form notes, however, may be difficult to work with, because important information could be located anywhere in the record: One provider may use specific methods or coding techniques not used by other providers. Therefore, it may be difficult to locate a specific piece of information,

Figure 10: Automated Records

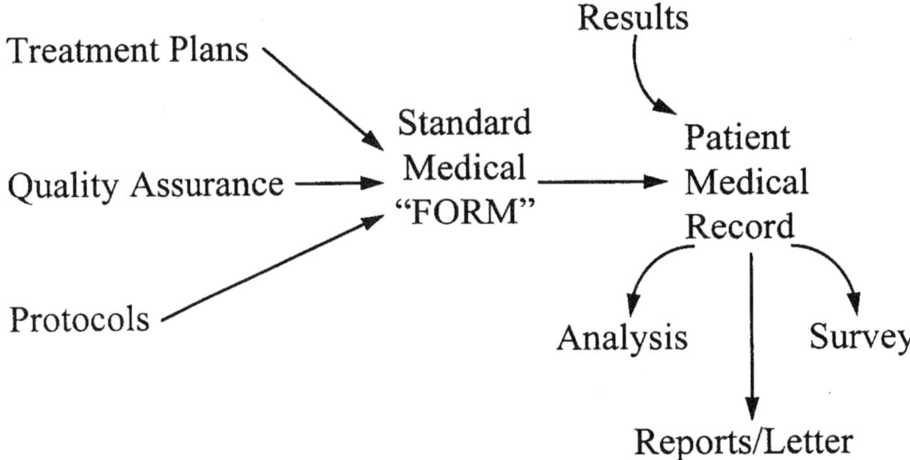

and a word search may not turn up all occurrences of a word because of abbreviations or inconsistent language.

Medical record systems will associate the free-form record with an incident of care. The medical record can be accessed through a diagnosis or a procedure code as well as through the patient. The integrated system will also control changes to the record by user and limit access to selected users.

Defined-Forms Format

A medical practice can define the group of information items that the operator will enter, as well as the information type (e.g., letters or numbers) and valid responses (e.g., ranges of numbers or a list of conditions). Providers will have to agree on the information to be included on the form and the order of that information and also will have to establish a policing mechanism to ensure that records are properly used.

Separate forms may be developed for a variety of diagnoses, problems, procedures, and patient profiles. For example, a practice may maintain separate medical forms by sex for newborns, children, and teenagers. If the practice is committed to forms, then providers will have to fill out a form for each appropriate patient service. Otherwise, any form-based analysis will not be reliable, as relevant forms would be missing.

Defined forms allow the practice to establish structure, but they do not allow for an elimination process or for jumping around in the medical record. For example, a practice may have one defined form for respiratory problems and another defined form for asthma. If the provider decides, in the course of filling out the asthma form, that another respiratory problem is the proper diagnosis, the information may not transfer easily to the appropriate form, and the provider may have to start over.

Knowledge-Base Format

Knowledge-base systems are built on top of thousands of diagnostic variables that may be combined into protocols or lists of diagnostic variables. The variables may be filled out on an ad hoc basis and cross-indexed with potential conditions, or the provider may fill out a complete diagnostic variable list for a particular condition. As the provider answers yes or no to the diagnostic conditions, the system may also ask for additional details. For example, an answer regarding a high temperature may be followed by a query for the actual temperature.

At any point in the process, the provider can jump to another protocol, and the previous answers will be reflected in the new form. All the clinical observations are associated with the patient's visit and may be cross-indexed to all the diseases in the knowledge base to identify potential courses of further analysis. The provider can also focus quickly on the protocol associated with a known condition and proceed from there.

Most knowledge-base systems were developed by a group of providers, who determined the diagnostic variables and protocols. The product is only as good as the developers of its protocols.

Language-Modeling Format

Language modeling enforces a sequence of responses to a medical record. The medical record is programmed to accept only a specific response to a query. Because the response is defined, the system will recognize only the expected response. For example, a medical record may address two aspects of a condition: frequency and severity. The system will accept only the words *hourly*, *every two hours*, *weekly*, or *monthly* for frequency, and *mild* or *severe* for severity.

Language responses can be modeled in any way necessary to get the appropriate information. They can be used in combination with the defined-forms format to support more effective voice entry.

ELECTRONIC MEDICAL RECORDS IN ACTION—TRACKING TREATMENT PLANS

Treatment plans add another twist to medical practice management. Under managed care structures, all providers will want to track treatment plans, for a variety of reasons:

- **To document quality** Treatment plans reflect the methods and protocols providers use to care for particular patients. Such standards may be established by various specialties, the medical practice, employers, insurance companies, and others.

- **To manage patients proactively to meet contractual requirements of wellness programs** Once the practice has committed to a patient wellness program, the system will need to support the activities of that program. The planning horizon for patient wellness could include a series of steps that follow patients throughout their lives; the need may be to address a temporary commitment. In any event, the treatment plan can be used as a trigger to solicit a patient visit, coordinate treatment plan activities with other patient services, and follow up on a cancelled appointment that was part of a treatment plan. Ideally, the system should allow the user to view the treatment plan for patient service, risk management, utilization management, and quality assurance perspectives as well as evaluate the plans within a user-defined time period.
- **To measure risk for committed treatments** In the course of treating patients, providers are constantly accumulating information on patient services that will be provided in the future. These incurred but not reported (IBNR) services can be used to quantify the exposure of the practice and to maintain more appropriate accounting records. Therefore, the treatment plan becomes a guide for patient services as well as a management accounting and practice management tool. The treatment plan should measure the projected value or cost of services the practice is committed to performing at a future date.
- **To manage provider time by identifying services to be provided but not scheduled** Treatment plans can be used to fill appointment slots while assuring that all contractual service obligations are met. For example, the practice could use the information gathered in the treatment plan to identify patients who are due for checkups or recalls and then schedule those patients during open appointment slots.

Treatment plans play a central role in serving patients. Treatment plans can offer a standard of care for numerous problems or continuing care standards, as follows:

- **A specific problem** A treatment plan would include a series of steps needed to resolve a problem. Each step could consist of a procedure code or action (e.g., a report to the insurance company, contact with a referring physician), a delay between steps in the plan, and a designated provider. A variety of standard treatment plans could be called upon and customized for each patient. For example, a pneumonia treatment plan could be called up and adjusted for the situation of a particular patient. The provider should also be able to enter a unique treatment plan according to the patient's needs. Note that the system should mark any steps that deviate from the standard treatment plans.
- **Continuing care** A treatment plan could be part of a standard wellness program, and the system could chain treatment plans. For example, new baby treatment plans could indicate visits once a month

for a year and then chain to a child plan that requires a visit every six months.

The treatment plan becomes a primary focus of the entire system. Outside referrals, patients' appointments, and various other functions are all part of the master plan for helping the patient. Physicians on a provider network in a multi-specialty practice could reference the treatment plans for a particular patient to track what other providers are doing with the patient.

Whether or not the treatment plan is the specific tracking mechanism, the more sophisticated practices must keep track of patient service, risk management, and practice management needs. The treatment plan option is useful for this because the plan links the patient's condition with all the activities and steps that have been defined as aspects of keeping patients healthy. Therefore, the practice can use a variety of automated tracking and management tools to manage patient services quickly and cost-effectively.

CHAPTER 7 • ELECTRONIC DATA INTERCHANGE

CONTENTS

7 ELECTRONIC DATA INTERCHANGE

One of the most onerous problems facing medical practices today is the avalanche of paperwork that must be exchanged with insurance companies, other providers, and patients. In many instances, reports and forms are printed off of one computer system and mailed, faxed, or hand-carried to another practice. The practice receiving the papers may enter important information or the entire contents of the forms into their computer system and file the information in the patient chart or some other paper file. Thus, exchange of information could be improved if there were some mechanism to transmit the information electronically between parties. Thereby, both practices may be able to cut down on the handling of paper and simplify access to information from multiple sources.

Achieving this basic objective requires dealing with a structural issue of medical care: Many services are initiated by one provider who refers the patient to other healthcare services. Electronic data interchange (EDI) may offer benefits to both the referring provider and the secondary provider (such as a hospital), but the first point of contact is where the initial information must be gathered and entered. This effort may not affect all providers equally. A primary care provider may send information on to other providers, but it is still the primary care provider who performs the initial data entry.

To cut the cost of handling paperwork, the larger players in the healthcare industry are establishing EDIs to move information from one provider to another and pass results and treatment information back and forth. Indeed, selected insurance companies and integrated delivery systems are requesting more electronic information from practices. A wide range of opportunities exists for exchange of electronic data that may benefit all concerns.

Here are some examples of uses of EDI:

- **Referral authorizations can be passed to a third-party administrator, who then sends them to an appropriate provider.** The authorizing provider's practice enters the referral into its system and passes the referral electronically, along with the patient's registration information, to the next provider or third-party administrator. When the patient calls that provider to schedule an appointment, the patient is already registered in the referred provider's system. Later, the referred provider's system may even check the referring physician's system to ascertain the status of the patient.

- **Providers can enter lab orders directly to medical labs.** A practice prints its own bar codes and label samples. When the test samples arrive at the lab with the appropriate bar codes and labels, the order information is already in the lab's computer, thus saving the lab sample preparation time. Also, there is less chance the lab will misread the order. The lab returns the laboratory results to the medical practice through a computer terminal. In many cases, the practice uses a software product provided by the lab to send the order and receive the results. Several practice management software vendors have similar products that load laboratory results into the medical records portion of their system.
- **Prescriptions can be entered into electronic systems for transmission to pharmacies.** The provider can enter the prescription information into the pharmacy's computer, so the pharmacy can have a prescription ready when the patient arrives. The provider can quickly determine a patient's current medications and can easily monitor usage and refills through its in-house medical records system. The in-house medical records system may also include a drug interaction monitor or maintain a drug formulary for patients in a managed care plan. The prescription history for the patient will be accessible to the provider for verifying patient treatments and drug histories.
- **Physicians can copy information about patients from hospital computers, and hospitals can accept certain requests for patient services through the computer.** The provider has access to the most current information and does not have to wait for it to be supplied by busy hospital staff. Specialists can quickly register patients who have been served in the hospital. Many hospitals are also developing strategies to enable them to act as a central repository of patient information within the local provider network. Under these structures, providers submit their treatment and patient service information to a central location for access by authorized providers.
- **Insurance companies can offer more information and faster payment to providers through a variety of electronic forms.** Existing insurers as well as de facto insurers (such as managed care plans through hospitals and employers) are demanding more information from providers in order to monitor patient care and costs. With EDI, a practice can verify payments and, in some cases, allow its own system to post electronic EOBs from insurance companies to patients' accounts, thereby minimizing the time required for the practice's staff to post insurance checks and provide the insurers with additional information at a reasonable cost.
- **Providers can receive inventory information from and place electronic orders with distributors of durable medical equipment.** Patients can quickly select the model or product they want and place an order from the physician's office. The physician office could also submit orders to maintain inventory in the practices and optometric shops.

In addition to providing the obvious benefits of eliminating paperwork, these organizations also seek a closer working relationship with physicians that they hope will evolve into more activity and more business.

If such a system is actively used, the traffic between providers will increase. The bigger the paper problem, the more use there is for electronic exchange of information. Insurance companies, hospitals, labs, and pharmacies are highly motivated to cut the volume of paper they send to and receive from providers.

These electronic data strategies do not necessarily produce efficiency at the level of the practice, however. The fact remains that, because the physician is the originator of requests for services from other providers, his or her office is the most logical location at which to capture the initial information and pass it on. Therefore, the practice has to fund not only the installation of front-end computer systems to capture the information and pass it on to the next step but also the operational costs of maintaining the information on a day-to-day basis. Be careful to insure that the practice derives the benefits from investing in medical software. For example, some lab systems are a poor investment because they can prepare the lab order but lack the tools to receive and graph the results.

Currently, most of the electronic relationships consist of a basic terminal or PC-based terminal package that allows the practice to submit information to or review information from another system. For example, a practice can submit an order to the lab and review the results later. The provider can also print out the results and file the test information with the patient's chart. Some systems will even store information locally and allow the provider to look up patient information as needed.

These systems still place a demand on the practice, because the same software does not contain information from all labs or hospitals. The provider may need to search several places to gather all information—the lab information is on the lab system, the provider notes are in the patient's file, and the billing information is in the practice management system.

Similarly, several insurers now allow practices to dial into their systems to check reimbursement rates and patients' eligibility. The actual reimbursement is transmitted either on an electronic EOB, which can be posted to the patient's account, or on a paper EOB, which the practice must manually verify to make sure the right amount was paid.

IMAGES

Issues regarding the movement of text-based information pale in comparison to those affecting the exchange of images. Images of forms, radiographs, and other pictures require thousands of times more disk space than a screen full of characters. A computer image consists of thousands of dots that the computer must track and manage individually. The exchange of images requires more sophisticated communications, security, and programs at each end in order to send the image, receive it, and attach it to the correct patient information records. Most products have yet to tackle the exchange of images among systems. Diagnostic-quality images can take up even more resources, because of the detail that must be transmitted and processed.

Several practice management software vendors can attach images to a patient record. However, many of these do not associate the image with clinical or treatment information. For example, a connection may not be maintained between an image and the date of service information. Many of these systems allow for various identification information to be associated with the image independent of the patient information. Examples of identification information may include user-entered dates, comment, diagnosis, source, and other data. Unfortunately, the identifying image information must be searched outside of the basic treatment and demographic information maintained by the system. If a user accidentally enters different identifying information about the image, it will be difficult to locate the image because the image cannot be accessed through the treatment record.

The basic intent behind exchanging information is to achieve more effective and efficient working relationships among the providers who serve a patient. For example, when lab tests and other studies are shared, everyone enjoys less paperwork. For that to happen, all parties must be able to send and receive electronic information, and a vehicle must exist to exchange information among the parties.

MANAGING EDI

Basically, EDI requires a phone line and an agreement between two systems about how information will be exchanged. Figures 11 and 12 illustrate the types of electronic relationships that providers are exploring. In Figure 11,

Figure 11: External Relationships Today

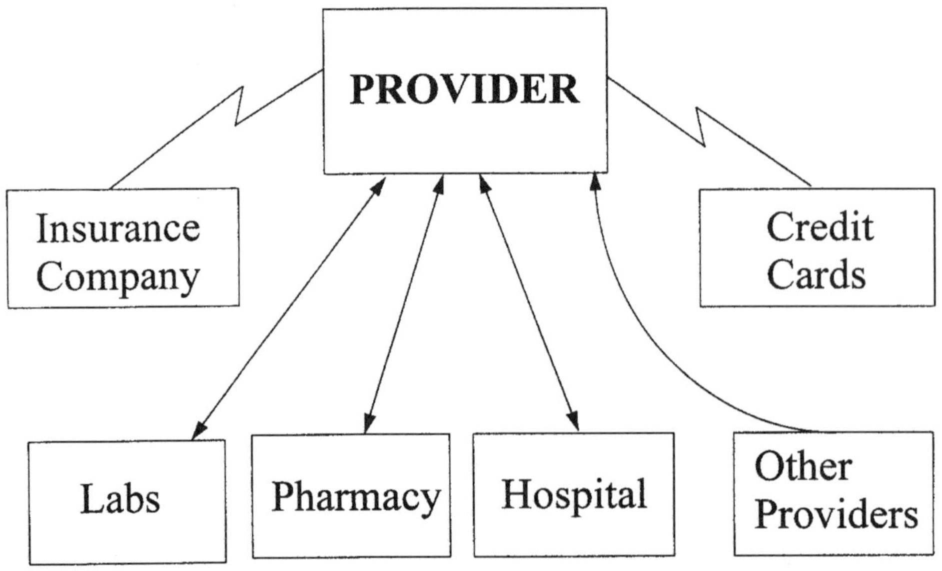

the practice has point-to-point relationships with each provider. In Figure 12, the practice passes all electronic data through a single point of contact.

Figure 12: External Relationships Tomorrow

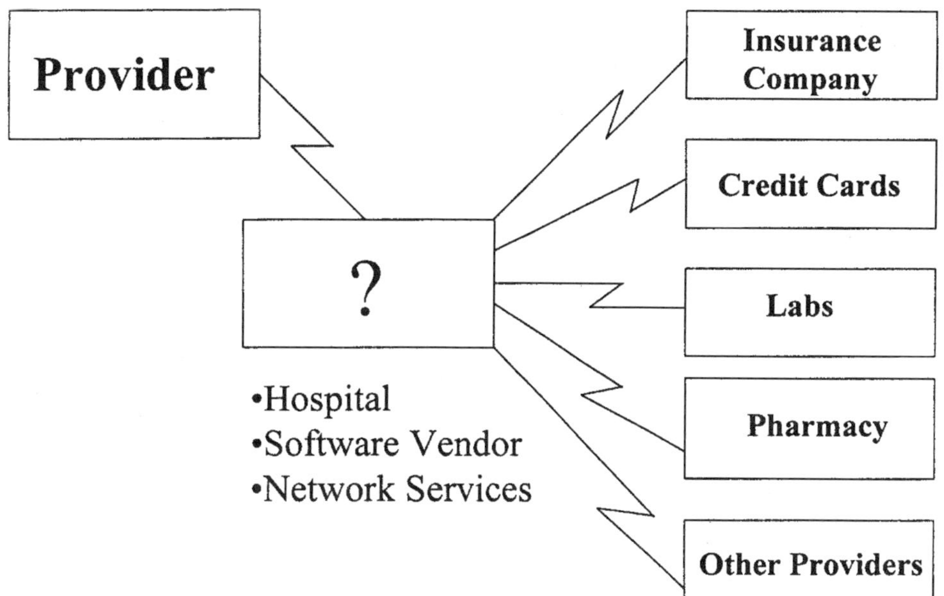

If a provider must personally work with each of the insurers, practices, pharmacies, labs, and hospitals with which it wants to communicate, there will be little time left for serving patients. The provider would have to contact each company and find out how it can communicate. Then the provider and the company would have to decide what information they want to exchange, and each entity would have to develop a mechanism to verify the other's data before adding the information to its own systems. Finally, each will have to find a place in its own system for the information. Someone will have to make sure that the two systems understand each other's information. If the definition of the information is even slightly off or the transmission even slightly corrupted, the computers will not be able to interpret each other's information properly, or, even worse, may initiate a process that will not help the patient. Larger organizations may require the provider to adhere to their way of exchanging information, regardless of the provider's needs.

Another option for lower volumes of information is to exchange information through a relay system. Relay systems use a PC as a terminal to initiate a session on Computer A. The relay system plays a script that queries Computer A for certain information, which is displayed on the screen. As the information is displayed on the screen, the PC captures the information according to a map of the screen that is displaying the data. Basically, the map associates a range of coordinates (row and column) with a name and stores the information on the PC. After all the information has been stored on the PC, the PC signs on to Computer B to "relay" the information to the second system. The script for the second system requests the creation of a record and fills in the fields interactively with the named data from Computer A. For example, the first name may have been the third field on Computer A, but the script "writes" the first name initially since that is the first field on the screen of Computer B.

Considering that the average provider may work with more than one hospital, several labs, a variety of pharmacies, and a large number of referring providers, coordinating electronic relations could become impossible for even large practices and smaller hospitals. The practice would have to develop, test, and maintain a separate connection with each of those other organizations.

To simplify this requirement, some players in the healthcare field are positioning themselves to act as a single point of contact for providers. Providers send all their data for electronic transmission to a single point, and that receiving service passes the information on to the other entities' computer systems. Those who propose to act as a communications switch include practice management software vendors, insurance companies, third-party information providers, telecommunications providers, and hospitals.

Practice Management Software Vendors

HBOC/Cycare, +MEDIC, and Physician Computer Network are examples of practice management software vendors that are actively working to become the telephone switch through which providers exchange information. In each case, information to be received or forwarded will be sent to the vendor's main communication switch location. The vendor will hold the information until the next time a communication takes place with the receiving system. If a response to the sending party is warranted, the receiving system will send back to the communications switch an acknowledgment or an answer to any request.

Currently, these services are limited to insurance claims and other basic business information such as credit card validations. These vendors would like to be a conduit for a variety of provider data to other providers, hospitals, labs, and others. For example, a provider may send a medical record to a specialist with the referral authorization.

Note that practice management vendors are focusing primarily on the exchange of text from one user of their system to another user of their system. They are not addressing the problems of sending information to other practice management systems or of exchanging images. Exchanging images requires a much larger capacity to move information. For example, while an electronic insurance claim may take up a few hundred characters of space, an image of an electrocardiogram (EKG) could take up several hundred thousand characters and a radiograph could require millions of characters.

Insurance Companies

A number of insurance companies already have electronic relationships with many medical practices. Currently, larger insurance companies accept claims directly from providers and allow those providers to log on to their system to check insurance eligibility, claim status, and even reimbursement amounts by CPT code. The insurance companies are actively working to expand their capabilities to maintain an active presence with providers. Some companies are working on referral authorizations and even communications with insurance service departments.

The large insurance companies have the capability and wherewithal to develop viable EDI networks, they have access to providers, and they are not committed to any particular practice management software or hospital information system; as a consequence, they likely will develop mechanisms to exchange data among practices with different software systems. Such a network would accept information from one software system and translate it into the format needed by another system. For example, if one system, sends out a file with an account number followed by a name, the target system needs to reverse the fields.

Third-Party Information Providers

A number of third-party information vendors offer standard insurance claim information as well as a number of practice support services. ENVOY/NEIC, Equifax, and HBO/CyData are examples of third-party information vendors that offer electronic claims, credit card validation, and check verification to medical practices. They are also seeking to provide data exchange options.

Third-party information vendors offer only information. They seek to funnel information into the systems of a variety of partners, so the vendors can market the information to end users and to the healthcare industry in general. For example, insurance validation information from insurers could be sold to providers.

Telecommunication Providers

A number of regional telecommunications companies are actively pursuing the healthcare market. Their objective is to act as a facilitator for images as well as to allow the general exchange of information. The exchange of images is particularly important to the telecommunications companies, because it takes advantage of new technologies and added-value services that are expected to generate significant future profits for the industry.

Although many industries could benefit from access to images, the healthcare industry represents a huge market that relies on a variety of images that must be shared among many people. The inability to share images can actually increase healthcare costs. For example, X-rays, lab tests, and EKGs may have to be repeated if the provider cannot review the image in another provider's records. If diagnostic-quality images could be reliably transmitted, such repeat tests could be avoided.

Hospitals

Hospitals are developing communication systems primarily to facilitate the exchange of information among the medical staff associated with that hospital. The hospital may also use such a system to provide infrastructure support to the physician–hospital organization. A number of hospitals are exploring initiatives that would enable them to take the lead in providing local healthcare and organizing regional healthcare groups.

Physician Networks

Physician networks include IPAs, PHOs, PPOs, and similar groups. Physician networks are interested in exchanging data to control costs and provide benefits to the provider base. Technology is particularly important to physician networks since computers are a key tool in supporting cooperative relationships (and exchanges of data) between a loose confederation of organizations. At the organization level, computers allow the network to capture information once and pass it onto the network quickly and effectively. Ideally, this would enable the network to respond more quickly to the needs of buyers.

THE INTERNET

More than 4,000 Internet sites have something to do with healthcare. Originally, the Internet was developed to facilitate the exchange of information among academic institutions. However, over the past few years, the Internet has exploded as a vehicle for commercial entities, governments, families, and individuals to gain access to information offered at various Internet sites or to offer information to all or selected users of the Internet.

Currently, most medical Internet sites offer a wide range of information. Internet sites are maintained by organizations, by hospitals, and by a host of practices, commercial suppliers, drug companies, and others. Some of these sources of information offer valuable data to providers and offer a forum in which to keep up with clinical issues as well as to maintain contact with people across the globe. Vendors offer ordering capabilities to their established customers over the Internet.

Internet information offerings are based on "hypertext." *Hypertext* consists of highlighted words within a document that are linked dynamically to additional information, to a query screen, or even to another Internet site. By pointing to a hypertext entry, the user can directly access another area or function or additional information. Hypertext products are also available on CD-ROM, so that accessing the Internet is not a necessity.

Outside of offering information, the Internet is a vehicle to exchange the various types of information discussed in this chapter as well as to comply with the requirements of the Health Insurance Portability and Accountability Act. (See Chapter 1, "Trends and State of the Industry.") A wide range of initiatives and products have been introduced in the marketplace to take advantage of the Internet in the healthcare field. However, many of these initiatives are in the early stages of offering practical assistance and support at the practice level. These initiatives will evolve rapidly when they become available.

Use of the Internet is affected by the following factors:

- **Communication infrastructure** The Internet offers a standard way to communicate with various sites of interest to the user. This vehicle presents a unique tool for research and access to current information. The general idea is that a practice would need only a connection to the Internet to contact and exchange data with a wide array of providers, insurance companies, hospitals, and research centers. In theory, the Internet offers cost-effective tools to allow all interested parties to access or interact with a specific site. However, a variety of healthcare organizations and vendors would prefer to serve the role of "phone system" to providers.

- **Security** One of the key problems facing everyone who is using the Internet is securing information. Many providers are concerned about allowing access to information through the Internet as well as tracking the use of information through the Internet. Organizations that are going to make highly confidential information available through the Internet will want to be able to maintain access logs as well as control over the security of that information. The available security mechanisms have evolved to address this issue adequately for many other applications. It is only a matter of time before these same mechanisms will be accepted by the healthcare community.

- **Software development** The development of a full range of software products that use Internet access effectively in the management of healthcare is still in progress. Development of Internet-based healthcare solutions is not so much contingent on development of the Internet as it is limited by the medical practice software vendors. Nonetheless, practices should seriously consider the strategies needed to provide data on the Internet as well as to access data from the Internet. Users should consider carefully the plans of their business partners (e.g., insurers, employers, drug companies, IPAs, and physician networks) to position their organization strategically to take advantage of Internet services as they evolve.

SUMMARY

All of these initiatives seek a way to facilitate the exchange of information among providers in order to cut down on paperwork and promote a network among healthcare providers. However, whoever owns the communication switch also controls access to the information and may be in a position to abstract information or control distribution. The business mechanism needed to ensure the final goal of an integrated healthcare delivery system is continuing to evolve.

CHAPTER 8 • ACCOUNTING ISSUES

CONTENTS

8 ACCOUNTING ISSUES

The integration of medical practice software programs with accounting is a highly significant undertaking. The vast majority of medical practices account for results on a cash basis. In the past, most practices were small and did not develop sophisticated accrual-basis tracking tools for either managerial accounting or financial reporting purposes. Indeed, many practices have deposit and payables activity that can be easily handled by such programs as Quicken or One-Write Plus.

Because cash-basis accounting requires a rather simple journal entry, most practice management systems did not develop links to download financial activity to general accounting software or did not create their own general accounting system. Medical practices are challenged by the most complex accounts receivable situation of any industry, but they have rather simple accounts payable and payroll. Few industries, for example, must explain themselves to the entity that is paying the bills of a second entity on the basis of the authorization of a third entity.

Older practice management systems addressed the receivables problem, but basic general accounting systems are too complex for the average medical practice. A practice that produces 100 checks per month does not need a complicated, multi-step invoice entry and check-printing process. A cash-basis practice that has only a few owners does not need complex general ledger posting and double-entry books.

Other developments are increasing the demand for more effective practice management and financial management tools. Risk-assuming practices are being challenged with problems not found in the fee-for-service environment, and larger practices are demanding more accountability and increased financial management. These challenges require that a practice use more analytical tools to manage its affairs and to ensure that funds will be available to meet future obligations. Indeed, simply pocketing the money left in the account after the bills are paid is not practical for larger practices with managed care risks.

The practice must have the tools to measure and manage future commitments, risk pools, growth of the practice, compensation plans, and costs in order to support managerial and financial accounting requirements.

FUTURE COMMITMENTS

Managed care providers often work under defined treatment plans that are specifically authorized by the primary care provider or the plan administrator. Primary care providers may treat patients for a problem that requires a specific recall sequence or a specific series of services. For example, a patient who has a chronic health problem may require tests every six months. Under fee-for-service or reduced-fee arrangements, these prospective services would generate additional revenue. If either the specialist or the primary care provider is capitated, however, these future services commit the practice to spending money from future capitated payments.

If the primary care provider covers the referred services, then the primary care provider will pay the fees of the specialist to whom a patient is referred. Future payments to other providers and out-of-pocket costs for future treatments represent future costs that should be recognized for managerial accounting purposes, if not for financial accounting purposes. If the entity is a cash-basis organization, the future obligations will have to be managed and monitored carefully.

Even if a cash-basis organization establishes a reserve for future services, a solid tax strategy requires that the "reserved" funds be distributed to owners at the end of the tax year. The cash-basis organization would find it difficult to leave the reserve in the practice, as this would increase taxable profits. Such organizations should seriously consider accrual accounting for tax purposes.

The reserve can be set aside according to one of several bases. A standard or reduced-fee schedule, or some cost basis, could be used to calculate the reserve. The fee basis should be applied to outstanding services, to calculate the total outstanding obligation and the reserve. Referrals to outside providers should be calculated on the basis of the outstanding services. Practices should be especially careful with outsider services, as claim submission may lag behind patient services. A service that was provided at the end of the month may not be billed until a few days into the new month. On a sophisticated system, the reserve and the cost of provided services could be calculated on the basis of the projected date of service for the referral.

The reserve should be set aside for an appropriate time in the future. The specific time frame will depend on the standard treatment window for the practice and on other business issues.

RISK POOLS

Many managed care plans establish risk pools to handle bonuses for underutilization or assessments for overutilization. The practice must be able to determine the bonus or payment independently and set aside reserves to cover any assessments. Similarly, bonus pool payments should be allocated to appropriate revenue classifications, periods in which the bonus was earned, and distribution accounts.

The bonus pool payment should be added to the payments from the plan to generate a true realization for the plan. The bonus pool can be affected by the efficiency of referring providers or by the plan itself. For example, effective patient wellness programs for one plan may minimize the services provided to plan participants. Similarly, for purposes of analysis, any assessment should be charged to the plan.

Both assessments and bonuses should be posted to the practice management system as well as to the accounting system to ensure that realization reports by plan will reflect all of the revenue and expenses.

LARGER PRACTICES

For larger practices, financial results must be available for a variety of offices, profit centers, departments, and areas of practice. To produce appropriate information, the practice management system must classify revenues correctly according to the appropriate distribution strategy.

Most practice management systems classify transactions by provider, location, and procedure code. Larger organizations also need reports on productivity and activity by department and profit center. If transactions are not classified by these factors then the system will not be able to generate reports based on a variety of factors. To support appropriate analysis, the system should provide trend reports over time and comparison reports with locations, providers, and departments in columns.

COMPENSATION PLANS

Currently, most practices pay providers a percentage of payments received—or whatever money is left in the checking account at the end of the month. For a variety of payment options being used today, however, direct payment credits may not be possible. For example, payments for capitation and a single payment for all services for a particular condition must be credited to providers differently.

The allocation of revenue to providers is as much a managerial decision as an accounting one. Distributing capitation payments on the basis of services rewards utilization of tests but does not reward provider efficiency. Because utilization increases costs, it would make sense for providers to be paid on the basis of patient wellness, appropriate use of resources, and effective treatments. Turning these concepts into an equitable compensation plan requires a variety of analytical reports and performance standards. Buying treatment slots, subcapitating providers for assigned patient panels, and reducing fee compensation are a few of the options.

COSTS

In the traditional fee-for-service environment, for many practices cost was not an issue. Reduced fee arrangements and risk-assuming capitated plans, on the other hand, place more responsibility on the provider to control utilization costs or to monitor costs to determine if a particular plan, provider, location, or service mix is profitable. In risk-assuming situations, such as capitated plans, patient services do not generate revenues; they increase expenses. Therefore, the practice is interested in the cost of providing services and in the relative efficiency with which various providers serve patients. Indeed, completing a variety of "standard" tests before a patient sees a provider may not be financially prudent.

Traditionally, medical practices have measured results by comparing payments received to the standard charge for each procedure code. New measurement tools and standards are needed for the managed care environment.

A variety of metrics are available to address this requirement. A practice could use a standard fee schedule or an expected payment to measure return on capitated plan or reduced fee arrangements. Some practices calculate the relative value units of the procedures to arrive at the payment per relative value unit. However, the real measure of performance should be the cost of a procedure.

Developing the cost of a procedure is a separate exercise, based on these various components:

- **Direct materials** Lab tests and in-office procedures have a direct material cost component.
- **Non-provider direct labor** By measuring non-provider labor costs, the practice can also evaluate the assignment of cost-effective resources to particular procedures.
- **Provider direct labor** Provider labor costs may be based on an imputed labor expense of a particular payment that will be made to providers for each procedure. The handling and measurement of provider labor should be connected to the practice's compensation system.
- **Patient administration and collections** Administration and collections expenses may be higher for more complex procedures if the preauthorization or collections process is particularly difficult.
- **Overhead** Overhead costs should be limited to particular expenses that are not easily applied to specific procedures. The overhead costs may consist of location-specific expenses, as well as practice-level expenses.

Once the costs for each procedure have been developed, the costs should be stored in distinct cost values for each procedure. The distinct cost values could then be applied to analyze the cost and margins produced by various classes of patients and plans. Note that the cost information may be produced by various methods, including activity-based costing.

Hard costs, direct staff costs, indirect staff costs, and provider costs are all reasonable measures for quantifying risk or measuring performance. Capitated payments could be reviewed in light of the added value of the procedure to the practice as well as the "gross profit" generated against hard costs. For example, if the hard cost of a lab test is $25 and the standard charge is $40, the added value to the practice is $15. The managed care contract may call for a $25 charge, whereas the practice may charge $30 to a capitated plan. The straight dollar realization process used by most medical software could be supplemented by an analysis that focuses on the money contributed to the practice. An HMO that represents patients who use many low-added-value lab tests would appropriately be compared with another plan that produces few high-added-value procedures. Objective analysis of the mix of services would provide a true performance measurement for the plan.

ACCOUNTING SYSTEM INTEGRATION

Most practice management systems are not integrated with accounting packages. Those that *are* generally pass a simple entry to recognize the receipt of cash and revenue. This basic entry may be generated for each provider separately as follows:

	Debit	*Credit*
Cash—Provider A	$1,000	
Revenue—Provider A		1,000
Cash—Provider B	$2,000	
Revenue—Provider B		2,000

These journal entries are passed to the journal entry posting file of the accounting system. To reflect the activity in the practice's books, the entries must be posted to the system through the accounting system's standard journal posting function. This strategy does not save much time, and the vast majority of current interfaces do not prevent changes to the journal entry before posting, which makes strong close procedures and paper audit trails a necessity. At a minimum, the daily sheet that documents the practice management generation of the journal entry and the accounting system journal entry posting register should be filed together in a posting log.

Once the journal entries are posted to the accounting package, the general ledger information and financial reports can be sent to a spreadsheet program, word processing program, or presentation product. These links are available with most commercial-grade accounting software products. The underlying practice management information can also be interfaced with spreadsheet programs, word processing packages, and presentation tools by generating a report file and the use of a report manipulation product (e.g., Monarch) or by abstracting the practice management information through a report writer program.

These basic interfaces will, of necessity, become more sophisticated in order to support more advanced business structures and more sophisticated financial analysis. As noted in earlier sections of this chapter, a variety of emerging requirements can be satisfied only by more effective accounting policies and tools. Regardless of the size of the practice, however, the practice receivables and management tracking tools will continue to generate the vast majority of accounting activity, while the accounts payable remain relatively simple.

To meet these requirements, the practice management systems will have to develop better cost accounting and managerial accounting methods, tools, and procedures. Future links could include the following:

- **Costing links** Classified standard costs for provided services will be passed to the accounting package. Actual costs could be posted to profit centers and cost variances could be tracked and monitored through the accounting system.
- **Inventory links** Procedures will be associated with a bill of materials to maintain inventory and recognize costs.
- **Compensation calculation** Revenues and direct costs will be posted to a separate profit center for each provider, so that provider compensation will be based on utilization and production. Amounts set aside for performance and utilization bonuses will probably be handled by journal entries.

Additional links are discussed in the section of this chapter titled "Future Commitments."

CHAPTER 9 • PURCHASING THE SPECIFIC PRODUCT

CONTENTS

9 PURCHASING THE SPECIFIC PRODUCT

Once a medical practice has determined what it wants a practice management software system to be able to do, it must select and purchase the specific products and modules to accomplish this. Because practices primarily rely on vendors for information on a product, the vendor's job is to make the software work for the customer and to ensure that the hardware base is powerful enough to handle the workload for the number of users. Since the customer may not be in a position to analyze the effects of a vendor's hardware recommendation, or a software work-around, the practice must be especially careful to examine fully how the software meets each requirement.

The first task in negotiating with a vendor is to develop a comprehensive list of everything the practice needs or wants to buy. What hardware and software are required to accommodate the new system?

HARDWARE

While hardware is often perceived to be one of the more confusing aspects of the system selection process, in actuality the hardware decision should be easily derived from the chosen software. Basically, hardware does the work according to "instructions" contained in the software. Hardware components perform a certain level of work in much the same way that a car is driven by a motor's connection to a drivetrain and ultimately to the steering wheel.

The vendor should be able to specify the computer system needed to handle the number of users and the volume of work the practice has indicated. More importantly, vendors should stand behind their hardware recommendations. Due to the continuing drop in the price of hardware, users should not be afraid to buy a more powerful system than the vendor recommends.

System size and speed are based on the number of users at any one time, the volume of patients, and the desired retention period for the information entered into the system.

1. **Number of users** Each user competes with other users for computer resources. Therefore, the system or systems chosen should be able to handle the total number of users reasonably expected to use the system at one time. Note that the workload on the system from a

single user can vary. Entering transactions will not use as many computer resources as printing a report. Most software vendors have hardware set up guidelines that identify the computing resources and memory needed to handle a set number of users.

2. **Volume of patients** The number of patients and transactions may have operational and processing effects on a system's performance. The vendor should set up the internal hardware components to handle the number of patients and the amount of associated data that the purchaser has indicated.
3. **Retention period** The longer the practice keeps information, the larger the files will grow. Each software product is based on a file structure that manages the information in the medical system. Some file structures can handle large volumes of information easily; others require periodic purging.

It would be reasonable to expect the hardware that is initially installed to handle all aspects of system operations for at least two years, and the practice should expect to use the software for at least five years. Even though hardware prices are bound to drop over that period of time, hardware upgrades take time and money. Someone must set up the new hardware, rearrange or move information to the new system, and verify that the upgraded system is operating properly. The system's standard of performance should be included in the contract, and the practice should have sufficient time to test the capabilities of the system.

The dynamics of the current computer hardware market guarantees that no matter what system is purchased, a cheaper and faster product will be available within 6 months. Many vendors and practices focus on hardware issues to allow for "maximum flexibility in the future." This approach is further complicated by vendors' continuing efforts to develop more advanced technology for use in their systems. Most vendors, however, do not have working versions of these new developments. Furthermore, a given practice may not have an interest in these developments or, more important, a gauge of how the practice might use such capabilities. The practice may be better off buying the technology it can use today. New technology options could be considered separately when they become necessary and when actual hardware and software are available for evaluation. For example, the purchase of voice recognition equipment could be delayed until a viable medical records strategy has been established and the necessary medical records protocols have been developed.

When sizing the system, it is better to err on the side of too much power. The relative cost of computer hardware has dropped so dramatically over the years that the cost of adding the incremental power required to give the operations of the practice some breathing room is not particularly significant. Indeed, saving a few dollars by cutting hardware may increase the time it takes to back up information or print bills.

Some software vendors do not sell hardware and refer practices to hardware suppliers with which they have a working relationship.

Frequently, a practice will seek alternative sources for hardware when purchasing a system, which works fine if the practice has a computer expert on staff. If the practice does plan to purchase hardware independently, assurance should be obtained from the software vendor that the software will work with the hardware. The user may ask the software vendor to include a statement in the contract that it has reviewed the hardware order and that the software will effectively work on the hardware. Similarly, the user should get some agreement on an independent hardware purchase.

If the practice lacks internal support, hardware should not be purchased independently. One practice bought hardware based on a discussion with the local superstore staff and ended up with overpriced equipment that didn't work with its practice management system.

SOFTWARE

Purchasing software is complicated by user charges and software module charges—and further complicated by a variety of usage-based and service fees. Several different fees are involved in purchasing software:

1. **Package fees** The basic practice management software package includes patient registration, patient billing, and insurance billing. Appointment scheduling, managed care, medical records, and electronic claims typically are available for an additional charge. The practice may purchase the entire package up front or allow for adding capabilities in the future.
2. **Database fees** Some systems accommodate many practices in a single system. Other systems require a separate database for each practice; these additional database charges can be quite substantial. The initial purchase agreement should account for additional databases for each company or practice served.
3. **User fees** User fees are charged on the basis of either the number of individuals using the system at a single time or the number of users who have access to the system. Concurrent-user charges are based on the greatest number of simultaneous users who will be on the system. If a practice is licensed for 10 concurrent users, an eleventh user will never be able to sign on. Charges based on the number of authorized users are based on the number of user IDs that are assigned to be on the system. If a user has an ID but never uses the system, the practice still must pay for the system use. In the Windows environment, many vendors base user charges on the number of stations that have the software loaded. Even if a PC accesses the practice management system for as little as five minutes a day, payment is charged for a full user license for that PC.
4. **Support fees** Support fees are annual, quarterly, or monthly fees that must be paid to gain access to training, problem resolution, and future releases of the product. Some vendors also offer multi-year

support contracts as part of the purchase price. The practice should avoid making any support payments more than a year in advance, because prepayment leaves the purchaser with little leverage in the event of a problem.

Regardless of the pricing strategy and mechanism, the user should be certain to develop a clear understanding of the cost structure and its effect on the purchase. If a particular situation falls outside of the standard pricing policies, the user should negotiate the price. For example, one vendor charged the first installation in each city the full cost of developing electronic claims relationships with the local Blues and Medicare. After working with the vendor, one of its customers was able to bring down the price to a more reasonable level.

CHAPTER 10 • CONTRACT TERMS AND CONDITIONS

CONTENTS

10 CONTRACT TERMS AND CONDITIONS

Once a product has been selected, the vendor and the practice must establish an equitable relationship. Vendors write their contracts primarily to lock the practice into an enduring relationship, but frequently the contracts do not address key issues that are critical to ultimate success. It is imperative that the practice read all the terms and conditions of the agreement. Many of these agreements include items that represent additional cost Contracts may include terms and conditions that could limit the flexibility of the use of the system. For example, many computer software contracts will not allow the license to be transferred if the practice is sold. The acquiring practice would have to pay the license fee again to acquire the software.

Vendor contracts vary widely. Some govern usage, access to the system, training, and support, while others are very limited with few specifics. In any event, an agreement should encompass the tasks needed to make the system useful and should form the basis for a continuing, results-oriented relationship between vendor and medical practice.

The practice must consider a wide range of issues and options when a system is being purchased and a contract drawn up, because each term of the contract could have an effect on the current operations and future options of the practice. For example, some vendors do not provide continuing education classes for new employee. The practice then would not have the continual support of the vendor in developing the knowledge and capabilities of the staff.

For most vendors, a proposed contract is the final step in the sales process. It generally consists of three parts:

1. **System purchase agreement** The system purchase agreement, which is made with the distributor or publisher selling the system, itemizes the equipment, software, and services that the practice is purchasing. The system purchase agreements should list all of the products and services included in the purchase. If something needed is not in the purchase agreement, a source for the item will need to be identified.
2. **Software license agreement** The software license agreement governs the terms and conditions under which the practice may use the software over the course of its relationship with the software publisher. Typically, the agreement is with the company that developed the software, and it includes a wide range of terms to control access to the system and secure the rights of the publisher. The software license usually includes terms that will affect the practice even if the system is replaced. For example, many contracts require a customer to destroy

operating copies of the software and documentation if it is no longer using the system.

3. **Continuing support agreement** The continuing support agreement sets up a relationship with the distributor or publisher to provide the practice with updates and to help resolve problems over the life of the system. The agreement also specifies the responsibilities of the vendor, the mechanism to request support, and how services are handled if the services fall beyond the service agreement.

Often, sections of these documents will be virtually identical to each other. In any case, the practice will want to ensure that each agreement clearly establishes the role of the vendor and the role of the buyer in the implementation process and manages the expectations of both parties throughout the life of the system. These agreements are discussed in detail later in this chapter.

In addition to these general business considerations, it is to the practice's benefit to see that specific issues are addressed in each agreement:

1. **Usage** The practice should be able to use the system as much as it needs to. For example, a practice should avoid a contract limiting use of the system to "regular business hours" when it is only practical for the practice to produce reports during other times.

   Another usage issue is how the practice will be affected by implementing new modules or similar changes. The agreement should spell out what it will cost to increase the number of users or make changes in the use of the software.
2. **Assignment** Because of the evolving nature of the healthcare industry, the practice will want to ensure that all rights and privileges can be transferred to new partners or sold to another party. Many agreements include clauses that prohibit the practice from assigning to or transferring to another party the right to use the software. If the software cannot be assigned to a new party, the practice may have to pay the vendor another licensing fee for the right to sell the business. Such a problem could deflate the value of the practice to the acquiring party.
3. **Additional purchases** If the practice expects to purchase additional modules, services, or rights to serve more users, the upgrade terms should be included in the contract. The agreement could include a specific price schedule, volume discount schedule, or an option to buy additional software at a certain date.
4. **Future developments** Every software company strives to enhance and improve its product. Typically, vendors make these enhancements available through their continuing support programs. However, many vendors are also working on the next generation of their product, which may have a different name or operate in a new environment (eg.., Windows or a Database Management System). These new products may not be provided to the practice under the support charges. The impact on the practice could be severe if the current

product were replaced by a new flagship product. If the vendor is developing such a product, the agreement should be structured to give the practice the right to buy the new product at a discount based on the current purchase. The contract should credit the practice for having purchased the current product if the practice subsequently chooses to upgrade to the new flagship product.

AGREEMENTS WITH VENDORS

System Purchase Agreement

The system purchase agreement specifies the components that the practice will purchase from the vendor. In most cases, the list of components will be meaningful only to someone who understands computers. Unfortunately, even someone who understands computers may not be able to determine if the hardware and modules can handle the practice's volume. Similarly, the initial installation of the system involves a variety of services. To avoid surprises as much as possible, the practice should be certain to cover all known issues and requirements in the purchase stage.

To help ensure that the system will be set up correctly, the practice should include in the agreement a profile of the volumes handled and a diagram of the location of various terminals and printers. Furthermore, the vendor should provide a detailed list of the hardware and components needed to run the practice. Following are some other important terms in the system purchase agreement:

- **Delivery and installation** The practice and the vendor should decide what "delivery and installation" means. Many contracts require payment as soon as the boxes of equipment are delivered. Unfortunately, the practice will not benefit from boxes of equipment piled up in the waiting room. Installment should be completed before payment is due.
- **Payment** Many vendors require a substantial deposit when the customer orders the equipment and the remainder upon delivery. Try to structure a deal that releases payments as the practice progresses. Key progress points include the following:
  - The system has been started and the software can be seen in action
  - The data from the old system can be called up on the new system
  - The employees have been trained
  - The practice is sending bills generated by the new system

  The practice should stipulate that final payment will be made when the system is actively supporting day-to-day operations.
- **Implementation** A projected implementation plan—with expected due dates—should be attached to the contract. The implementation plan assigns tasks and supports the scope of the contract. The practice should have a clear idea of its own level of effort and what it may expect from the vendor. Set-up formulation, data conversion,

modifications, installation, and activation should be covered in the implementation plan. If the practice has several sites or is purchasing several modules, intermediate goals should be established for the vendor and the practice. This will enable the practice to gauge success and progress more easily.

- **Training** The agreement should specify a comprehensive training plan for the initial installation as well as more extensive training for key users. The practice should also set up an accommodation for training future employees. If the vendor imposes a limit on training, make sure that the amount of training will be able to serve employees adequately. Training will be needed for the staff to get going, and follow-up training will be needed on more advanced features. The training location should be specified. Ideally, the staff should be trained in the vendor's office. Training will achieve greater results without interruptions and distractions.
- **Modifications and enhancements** Any upfront modifications or add-ons should be specified in the original contract. Expected changes that the practice knows it will want should be part of the complete purchase agreement. The costs of the changes should be itemized in the contract. The practice should be guaranteed the opportunity to verify that the custom components work as agreed by testing the customized features as well as any other programs that may have been affected by the changes. For example, a special end-of-month process to calculate physician compensation from payments should be verified against the end-of-month activity report.
- **Confidential information** Most vendor contracts stipulate that all of their information on the product and software is considered confidential. The agreement may limit the buyer from showing the system to others or even keeping a log of the employees who have access to the system. These types of terms are impractical and bothersome. On the other hand, the vendor should not disclose any information about the practice without written permission from the practice. One vendor agreement stated it could disclose information that became public knowledge. In other words, if a patient showed up on the cover of a tabloid newspaper, the vendor could comment on the fact that person was a patient of its customer. Obviously, that term was not acceptable.

Software License Agreement

The software license agreement may be with a company that owns the software and uses the vendor as a distributor. In other words, the practice may buy a system from a vendor but be required to sign a software license agreement with yet another company that is actually the publisher of the software.

The software license agreement is often portrayed as just a bit of paperwork that is a standard contract. However, the practice does not have to sign such an agreement as is, and would be well within its rights to obtain clarifications and necessary changes by working directly with the company that owns the software. The following issues should be considered in formulating a contract:

- **Copyright protection** The vendor should protect the practice from any claims of copyright infringement. Unfortunately, many contracts give thc publisher the right to take away software if an infringement suit is brought and the publisher chooses not to defend itself. This means that the other party to an infringement suit against which the publisher chooses neither to defend itself nor to offer a settlement could walk into a practice and remove the software, rendering the data, hardware, training, and support investment worthless. The vendor should promise to defend itself or to put forth its best efforts to arrive at an amicable resolution.
- **Retention of materials after lapse of license** Most system contracts require that any and all materials be returned to the vendor when the practice stops paying support fees or stops using the system. However, due to recordkeeping retention requirements, data on the old system may need to be accessed long after the practice has stopped using the system. Ideally, the practice should be able to keep the system intact with one or two terminals for reference purposes. The practice will also want to keep the documentation as a reference source for future research on data in the system or for interpreting reports.

Continuing Support Agreement

A continuing support agreement defines the scope of continuing support that the vendor will provide to the practice. At a minimum, the practice should insist that any continuing support agreements include phone support to answer questions and troubleshoot, free upgrades of the purchased software as they become available, debugging of errors in the software, and repair of equipment that breaks down. Some vendors also offer remedial training for existing employees and initial training of new employees.

Consider the following key continuing support agreement issues:

- **Standard of performance** The contract should state how quickly the vendor will respond to problems. Most vendors respond on the basis of the severity of the problem. A request to repair a broken-down terminal will not be treated with the same urgency as a message that the practice's file indexes have been corrupted.
- **Continued access to the software** Some vendors require the practice to make continuing support payments in order to maintain a system license. If this is a condition of using the system, the resulting cost should be considered when the practice is still in the stage of comparing products. Other contracts are a lease for using the software for a specific period of time. For example, one vendor sells a lease for five years. At the end of five years, the customer would have to buy a new

five-year license. Depending on the situation and needs, lease arrangements may not be acceptable and should be considered carefully.

- **Warranty** The software should be warranted to be free of defects during the warranty period. The document should also identify a written document as the reference for determining if a problem exists. For example, a software user's manual could be used as a performance standard for the warranty.

LEGAL REVIEW

Once the vendor and the practice have worked out all the business terms and conditions of the purchase, a competent, independent legal resource should review the contract. Although an attorney may not be familiar with the business issues or the technical intricacies of the project, he or she can provide a valuable check that the contract does not contain hidden legal problems that could hinder the practice later. For example, a vendor may not feel compelled to resolve a problem if there is no penalty for failure to perform or if the amount of the penalty is trivial.

CHAPTER 11 • IMPLEMENTING THE SYSTEM SUCCESSFULLY

CONTENTS

11 IMPLEMENTING THE SYSTEM SUCCESSFULLY

Implementing a medical computer system requires a great deal of planning, because a new computer system will affect everyone who comes in contact with the medical practice. Acquiring a new computer system is also an opportunity to examine the role that clinical as well as administrative practices can play in improving operations and controlling costs. Unfortunately, few practices have the resources to support and control the installation and implementation processes fully and comprehensively. All practices, however, have staff who understand what needs to be done and who are the real keys to ensuring the success of the project. For example, the practice could set up teams of internal staff to handle the details of the implementation process under the guidance of an outside resource.

STEPS FOR SUCCESS

Here are five basic steps to installing and implementing a new computer system successfully:

- Instituting appropriate policies and procedures
- Setting up hardware
- Setting up software
- Converting data
- Training

Instituting Appropriate Policies and Procedures

For Office Operations Generally

The key to any implementation process is to institute policies and procedures that take full advantage of the practice's investment in computers and meet the practice's service and business objectives. The typical medical practice operates using methods that have evolved over time, and few practices ever seriously examine how their methods affect the practice overall.

As a practical matter, current policies and procedures should be evaluated over the entire course of the software selection process. Then, after a product has been selected and is being installed, the practice must revise and develop the specific procedures that will make its investment produce results.

Most computer software is written to handle a wide range of practices. Products use parameter tables and master files to control how the system looks to the practice. Parameter tables have switches which turn various options on and off and control processing. For example, a parameter table may contain the aging categories for the aging report or it may contain the default to use at charge entry. Master files contain selections that are used to enter patient information and charges. Insurance companies, patient types, and procedure codes are examples of master files. How these software options are set up will impact how useful the system is and how pleased the user will be with the results.

A practice should consider carefully each decision concerning setting up the system. The reasons for each decision should be clear and all of the factors that affect the practice should be weighed. A decision based on the current system may not be the most beneficial in the future. The new system will work differently from the old system.

The practice should critically review every aspect of its administrative and business operations. Old policies and procedures should be revised, or even discarded, and new ones should be developed to cover every step—from scheduling a patient appointment to receiving final payment. This process will result in changes to staff functions, job descriptions, and the way the office works. These efforts are referred to collectively as "re-engineering the workflow."

The vendor may recommend something because other clients use it, but each buyer should evaluate what is best for its own practice. Each practice has a different mix of services, payors, and patient relationships to manage. The practice should be wary of vendors who suggest leaving everything as is and making changes ad hoc. Such a strategy will only delay any positive results.

For the New Computer System

In addition to office operations, computer system policies and procedures should be reviewed.

First, given the critical role that the newly purchased computer system is meant to play in supporting managed care issues, the practice needs to ensure that proper backups are regularly maintained so that the practice can continue to provide service in the event of a system loss.

The primary prevention measure is to buy a system that provides some level of protection against loss resulting from hardware failure or damage. Depending on the role of the system, protection may cost anywhere from a few hundred dollars for an emergency electrical power supply to thousands of dollars for back-ups to key system components. For example, a "mirrored" disk will allow the system to continue to operate in the event of a disk failure, because the second disk duplicates the contents of the first disk. If one of the disks fails, the other disk will continue to operate.

System back-ups should be performed daily, and separate electronic back-up files should be available to cover at least a two-week rotation. In other words, at any point in time, the practice should be able to restore the system to the way it was two weeks before. Also, the current back-up should be stored at another site. Local copies of the back-ups should be stored in a fireproof safe.

Further, the back-up tapes should be secured at all times, because the treatment and medical record information stored on them is confidential.

As long as the patient and practice information is properly backed up and secured, the practice need only consider what would be required to replace some or all of the hardware if the system failed. A defective printer, terminal, or other peripheral can be supported simply by buying an extra device. The extra terminal or printer can immediately be swapped with the problem device.

Consider the impact of a catastrophic loss of the practice's main computer system. It is possible to ensure emergency replacement by setting up a contract with a disaster recovery service. A disaster recovery service offers a similar system setup that the practice can use if the entire system is lost. Note that PC-based local area networks (LANs) can be replaced easily, while some mini-computers take longer to replace.

Setting Up Hardware

In most cases, the vendor will configure and set up the hardware. The hardware should be loaded and tested before it is delivered to the practice.

The actual installation at the office should be completed a few days before the system is intended to be used for training or initial file loading.

The hardware should be set up based on the newly established policies and procedures and on the role the new computer system will play in the practice. For example, if the system is used mainly for billing, losing the system for a few hours will not affect the practice dramatically. But if the system is used for scheduling or for maintaining medical records, loss of the system could inconvenience patients and prevent providers from serving them. If a system has a large number of users, a shutdown could cost the practice significant time and money.

A number of environmental and installation protections can be put in place to protect the practice from such problems. An uninterrupted power supply, limited access to the computer location, and computer hardware that can tolerate different types of breakdowns are examples of ways the system can be protected.

This last example, system fault tolerance, guards against system failures by providing redundant components to compensate for different system breakdowns. Fault-tolerant systems consist of two completely operational systems, one of which will take over if the other fails. Thereby, one of the systems can become disabled with few interruptions to end users. Thus a fault-tolerant system can continue to operate in the event of a complete failure of any component.

High-availability systems provide redundant components for the parts of the system that have a relatively higher chance of failure than other parts of the system. High-availability systems typically include protection for disk drives and the power supply. They also include side-by-side redundant components inside the system. For example, a high-availability mirrored disk system includes two side-by-side disks that store the same information. If one disk fails, the second disk still operates. Another type of high-availability system includes duplicate connectors and disk interface cards.

When weighing what a system loss could cost its operation, the practice must be sure to consider what the system will be used for and who will need to access it. If the system supports several sites, many users, or critical services (e.g., medical records, patient flow), the practice should seriously consider investing in a high-availability or fault-tolerant option to add another measure of protection.

Setting Up Software

All software packages have system setup tables and parameters that allow the software vendor to change the operation of the software to meet particular needs. Setup parameters can include a wide range of options, and the practice will have to decide what issues it needs the software to address, from the amount of time to allow for a typical appointment to the text of the messages on bills that have older balances.

The software setup should be based on the expectations of the practice and not on its current methods. The software setup must also support the newly established policies and procedures. Deferring setup issues until after the system is set up will cause problems later. For example, if a coding method is changed after the system is used for a couple of months, management reports will reflect the change in coding and the results could be inconsistent.

Many software vendors combine the initial training effort with the software setup task. Other vendors base the software setup on several meetings that take place before training begins. In either case, the practice or users must answer questions that will guide the way the system is set up and ultimately used. In fact, the answers to various setup questions will guide how literally hundreds of software options and dozens of fields will be used. The practice must guide the vendor in every aspect of setting up the system, from how the router will print and look to whether an insurance write-off is posted automatically or manually

Some systems include software setups that can be managed only by the vendor or distributor; other systems allow all options to be maintained by the practice.

Several kinds of software setup needs will arise, including the following:

- Parameters, the switches that turn various software options on or off
- Master files, which contain the basic information used to organize and control the system

- Run-time options, fields that allow the user to produce different reports by changing the sort order, totalling, or records included in processing

Parameters

Parameters are also called policies, options, drivers, and variables. Some parameters cannot be changed after setup, while others can be changed at will. For example, some systems have a switch that determines whether accounts will be tracked on an open-item or balance-forward basis that cannot be changed. Other systems allow the setup of default codes, which speeds data entry because they can be changed as often as desired.

Note that parameters may be found in the master files in one system or as a run-time parameter in another system. For example, billing cycle definitions may be a standard set of billing rules for the entire system, a master file record that can establish a variety of billing rules within the same system, or information that is entered in the billing selection screen when billing is being processed.

Any parameter that cannot be easily changed should be reviewed closely. Each parameter selection has both obvious and subtle effects on system utilization. For example, a system-wide default office for posting charges may be useful for a single-office practice, but a separate default office for each user may be more effective for multi-office operations.

Typical parameters include the following:

- Transaction tracking, to govern the handling and posting of charges and payments—with options like payment posting—and to display orders such as FIFO, LIFO, and open item.
- Operational defaults for processing, such as standard appointment schedules, and entry defaults. Entry defaults include charge, payment, and patient registration defaults. Initially, the defaults are used to fill the entry screens and can be overridden by the user. Access controls govern the user's ability to access data and functions. Some systems allow security to be assigned at the menu level, while others control specific functions (e.g., entry or deletion) within the system.

Master Files

Master files contain the key reference information that will be used to enter information in the system. Master files include providers, locations, service codes, adjustment codes, and payment codes. Some systems also include ZIP codes, patient classifications, billing cycles, and other information.

Master files are used to standardize information throughout the system—to ensure consistency and to support various management reporting options. Many master files also include categories or summarization codes that can be used to summarize activities for management reports. For example, a procedure category may be used to summarize office visit procedure codes on activity analysis reports.

Master files are dynamic and will be built continuously over the life of the system. For example, infrequently used insurance companies will be added from time to time. Procedures should be established to avoid adding more than one master file record for the same item.

However, procedures should be set up to insure that new records are generated and that these new records are set up in a consistent fashion. Many practices lose control of insurance company files because front desk operators have difficulty finding the correct insurance record. In many cases the operator may enter in a company that is already in the file under an abbreviation (ex. PA instead of Pennsylvania) so that one company has duplicate entries. Another problem arises with the use of the word *the*; some operators will enter the word and some will eliminate it, if the staff is not given clear instructions on practice policy.

Run-Time Options

Run-time options include processing and reporting selections—such as providers, offices, service dates, and procedure codes—that the user makes as the program is started. Run-time options can be made more useful by combining them with a job scheduler or the ability to save the information. Saved information allows the practice to recall previously selected report or production options. Job schedulers allow the practice to define standard times and options to run specific reports. For example, an aging of all accounts over 60 days could be produced automatically every Monday morning.

Run-time options can be changed easily as the needs of the practice evolve. Parameter changes and master file changes can substantially affect the system's operation and results. For example, changing a patient classification code may result in management reports that are not comparable with previous results.

The system setup has a variety of long-term implications for the practice. Indeed, even initial results of the coding and operational preferences in the system setup may not be known for several months. The original list of requirements should be examined closely in light of possible long-term implications, to ensure that the setup makes optimal use of the system as well as to reflect the practice's operational and management objectives.

Converting Data

If the practice is already using a computer system, the information may be sent electronically from the old system to the new one, or the information may be entered into the new system manually from old system reports. If the practice currently has no computer, information must be entered into the new system manually from existing ledger cards or account information.

Although the goal is a worthy one, along the way are serious pitfalls to undertaking an electronic conversion. One of the key concerns during any implementation process is to minimize disruptions to the practice and its patients. Disruptions could include incomplete bills, delays in billing, delays in filing claims, and failure to post appointments.

Before embarking on electronic conversion, the practice must answer the following questions:

Is the current information reliable and accurate?

Practices sometimes change systems because they lack confidence in their data or have other problems with their current system. Frequently, this lack of confidence can be traced to a particular event or point in time. One group, for example, traced its data problem to when the practice started posting EOBs on an open-item basis. In other situations, the data is not reliable because of office policies and procedures. For example, a practice that does not file insurance claims for its patients may have dated or incomplete records of patients' insurance coverage. Such a practice would be better off not converting its data electronically.

If staff are not confident of the data, then they should seriously consider a manual conversion. Whether the conversion is manual or electronic, however, the office staff will have to compile and verify the information carefully to minimize the entry of incorrect information into the new system.

Is enough information available to convert?

Some vendors push electronic conversions in order to let the practice benefit from the vendor's previous experience. However, electronic conversions are not necessarily the most cost-effective ones. A typical electronic conversion can cost $5,000, but a manual conversion can run approximately $1.50 per patient. Practices that have 2,000 active patients may be able to enter active accounts more easily and economically by hand.

In making this decision, the practice must consider the net usable information. Patients who have not been in contact with the practice for more than a year or who do not have an outstanding balance should be eliminated from the conversion process.

Can the vendor convert the data from the old system to the new system?

Some vendors consider data conversion a puzzle they would like to learn to solve. If the vendor has not previously converted from the package the practice has chosen, using another conversion option or another vendor is a worthwhile consideration. The vendor would have to practically reverse-engineer the existing system to successfully convert the data. For example, some systems maintain audit trails using special keys and linking information that cannot be deciphered easily.

Before planning a data conversion, the practice must consider the types of data conversion that should be done:

1. **Master files** Master files, which include ICD-9 codes, CPT codes, and providers, are the heart of any system and should be reviewed carefully. They are also the files that drive a variety of features. Because most buyers are changing to a system with more features than they had before, the master files will probably have the greatest number of new fields to be set up. Electronic conversion may provide few benefits.
2. **Demographics** Demographic conversion transfers patient information but not financial transactions into the new system. Demographics are relatively easy to convert, because there are no accounting issues to deal with and few audit problems.
3. **Balance forward** Balance-forward conversion brings over the remaining balance on a patient account. Regardless of how many services, visits, or payments are reflected in the balance, only the total balance is converted to the new system. Therefore, it is impossible to tell why the patient owes money or to post payments on an open-item basis.
4. **Open item** Open item conversion brings over each outstanding charge and the underlying payment and adjustment information that resulted in the outstanding amount for that charge. Open item conversions are particularly tricky, because systems can differ dramatically in the level of detail they maintain. Some open item systems track only the outstanding amount of the charge and not the activity that resulted in the current balance. If the new system cross-indexes the charges with the applicable payments, the conversion process would have to include logic about which charges to post a payment to. Without a historical record of how charges were paid, matching charges to payments would be a guessing game.
5. **Historical information** For the practice to retain access to complete information, all of the historical information could be converted to the new system or the old system could be kept active until the practice no longer needs data from it. The practice will have to balance the cost and effort of converting information from the old system against the cost and inconvenience of maintaining the old system as a reference source.

Whether the practice already has an computer system or is converting from a manual system, several steps must be completed to support the conversion effort:

1. **Document the mapping of data from the old system to the new system.** The practice should develop a document, for use by the vendor and staff, that shows where data from the old system are to be placed in the new system. The document will guide manual conversion efforts or serve as a standard by which to measure and verify the conversion effort.

2. **Test the data conversion.** The vendor should be given a test "dump" of data from the old system to convert. Since the vendor is ultimately responsible for loading the data into the new system, the practice should consider assigning the conversion efforts to the vendor. This way, the practice can concentrate its efforts on the *accuracy* of the conversion. The practice should review the effectiveness of the conversion and verify the data map. If the conversion is a manual one, the test will help ensure that the staff understand where to obtain the information and where to enter it into the new system.

Training

The training plan must address the operational and personnel issues that prompted the practice to seek a new or revised system. Training consists of teaching users the mechanics of the system as well as clarifying any changes in procedure or strategy. The software vendor is the best candidate for training users on the capabilities of the new system. Practice supervisors and managers can concentrate their efforts on how the system will be used on a day-to-day basis.

Training typically covers three main topics:

- System setup
- Daily activities
- Reports

1. System setup training involves exposing users to the various system options. By the time training starts, the system setup should be established. The practice should be careful to inform users of how the system is set up, but it should also train efficiently, by limiting the amount of time spent on unused system options. Knowledge of unused system options could confuse new users.
2. Daily activities training covers the daily uses of the system, from scheduling to charge entry to billing. In larger offices, users may be limited to a particular set of tasks. For example, centralized schedulers may use only the appointment scheduling portion of the software. All practices, however, should attempt to cross-train users to provide backup staff and to sensitize users to the impact their work has on the practice.
3. Reports training is an evolutionary process. In some cases, reports may not be useful for more than a year after the system is in use. In other cases, transitional issues may complicate the preparation of standard reports for several months after the system is installed. Initially, users should be trained on using the reports that will be needed to audit and reconcile the system on a daily basis. Additional training to review management and analysis reports should be scheduled at three months and again at one year.

During training, all the system options that were requested and have been programmed into the software are presented. The practice may want to limit system setup training to supervisors, who can decide how best to use each aspect of the system. For example, the software may divide procedures by area of service, but management would know what areas of service to include and how to classify procedures. In a separate, later training session, nonsupervisory users could be trained on the specific issues they deal with on a daily basis.

Training can be performed in a variety of ways. To introduce the staff to the basic operation of the system, videos and computer-based training tools can be used instead of a vendor representative, and therefore when time permits rather than in a formally scheduled session. Any training tool can include information that will not be used by every user, but all users can profit from a better overall understanding of the system infrastructure.

Classroom training at the vendor's location would minimize interruptions to the practice and allow staff to focus intensively on learning the new system. If the practice is large enough, or the software is significantly customized, the vendor may design a training program specifically for the practice.

Additional training time should be scheduled to support system activation. Having an experienced trainer on-site and available to users is critical during at least the first few days the system is used.

ACTIVATION

Once the installation and training efforts are complete, the practice should start the system activation process—the first use of the new system and the migration of activities from the old system to the new one. The activation process can begin only when all of the hardware installation, software setup, training, and data conversion have been completed and verified. If users are not familiar with operational changes, or if data conversions cannot be verified, then activation of the new system should be delayed.

Some practices will run the old manual or electronic system and the new electronic system concurrently before fully activating the new system. The benefit of concurrent, or parallel, operations is that the practice has a fallback if it encounters problems with the new system. The purpose of concurrent processing is to verify the operational integrity of the new system. The cost of parallel operations is that for a time the workload of the staff will double.

For the system to operate on a parallel basis, information must be entered on both systems daily. Ideally, the results are the same on both systems. In reality, the practice must establish a reasonable expectation of what constitutes "the same results." The new system was implemented because of problems or deficiencies in the old system. The new system may use new coding methods, operational procedures, and processes. Comparability may be limited to just a few areas. For example, a practice may verify only the charge amounts and receipts on a daily basis. Appointment scheduling may not be verifiable, because the practice formerly used a schedule book without collecting treatment or referral information. Once the practice is comfortable with the new system, operations on the old system can be discontinued.

FOLLOW-UP SUPPORT

Once the system is in use, the practice should fine-tune issues as they are encountered and review overall performance periodically, thereby maintaining the relevance of the system and the applicability of the practice's policies and procedures.

It is also important to maintain an active continuing training program to improve staff knowledge of the system in use, as well as to keep abreast of developments in the product and the medical software industry. Advanced user training and user group meetings will expose the staff to the insights of a broader range of users and situations, bulletin boards, advisory committees, and release notes.

APPENDIXES

CONTENTS

APPENDIX 1 • BASIC PRACTICE ASSESSMENT

I. General Information

Company Name: ______________________ Date: ________________

Address: ___________________________ Phone: _______________

___________________________________ Fax: _________________

City/State/ZIP Code: ____________________________________

Type of Practice: _______________________________________

Business Status: Corporation____ Partnership___ Sole Practitioner____

II. Staff

How many employees do you have? Full-time:______Part-time:______

Physicians:_______ Physician's Assistants:_______ Nurses: _______

Technicians:______ Office Management:_______ Front Desk: _______

Transcription:________ Billing/Insurance:_______ Accounting:______

Other: ____

____

III. Offices

How many locations do you have? (If more than one, list below.)

Location	*Days Open*	*Patients per Day*

IV. Services Offered

Office Only:_________ Hospital Services: _________

Laboratory Services:_________ Radiological Services: _________

Other:____

____

V. Key Issues

What are your current concerns with computerizing your practice?

____

____

____

____

What are your expectations of the computer system?

____

____

____

____

List the three most important tasks you want the computer to handle:

____

____

____

____

VI. Daily Activities

How many patients are seen daily?_________

How many payments are received daily?_________

How often are patient bills sent?_________

How are patients referred to the practice?

____

____

____

Describe the current charge and payment posting process:

____

____

____

VII. Insurance/Billing Information

List the major insurance plans you deal with and the estimated practice volume:

Top three commercial insurance carriers:

__________________________ ______%

__________________________ ______%

__________________________ ______%

Top two HMO/PPO plans:

__________________________ ______%

__________________________ ______%

Top two capitated plans:

__________________________ ______%

__________________________ ______%

Medicare: ______%

What is the current payment policy?______________________

____

Average number of procedures per patient:______

Average monthly A/R aging: _______

Number of bills sent per month:_______

Claims filed per month:_______

VIII. Computer/Systems Information

In the following areas, what improvements would you like to see from the new system?

Patient scheduling/Recalls:

____

____

Billing:

____

____

Collection:

____

____

Practice analysis:

____

____

Patient/Treatment management:

____

____

Medical records management:

____

____

Word processing:

____

____

Spreadsheet:

____

____

What software packages have you looked at?

____

____

____

What obstacles have you experienced in your efforts to automate?

____

____

____

Collect copies of the following documents to compare with the potential packages:

Practice brochure
Office procedures
Appointment book page
New patient intake form
Fee schedule
Patient ledger card
Super bill
Insurance form
Statement
Deposit slip
Day sheet
Collection notice
Recall notice
Management or accounting reports

APPENDIX 2 • SAMPLE FUNCTIONAL LIST OF NEEDS

General

Has online help

Limits user access to specific functions

Produces audit trail of transaction entries and master file updates

Practice Operations

Assigns action items and ticklers for a patient account to users

Provides messaging and ticklers with author, type, and date information

Accepts schedule of reports to run at user-specified time and frequency (e.g., daily, weekly)

Scheduling

Supports wave scheduling by appointment type for providers, labs, and X-ray

Allocates time based on a template for designated appointment type (e.g., comprehensive medical exam)

Allows online verification of patient name, address, and insurance over phone before scheduling an appointment

Allows online review of account and recording of payment commitment at scheduling time

Schedules multiple resources at one time (e.g., labs and X-ray)

Manages providers at multiple service locations

Easily maintains schedule changes: bumps, cancellations, and no-shows

Allows schedule details at procedure-code level with a check against authorized procedures on referrals. Such procedures can be scheduled in only the appointment slots designated for that appointment type.

Requires minimum information for new patient appointment scheduling

Easily identifies new patients on the daily appointment sheet

Customizes router by provider and appointment type

Can tag patients at arrival and departure

Produces an appointment sheet by provider

Produces a management report by scheduled procedures, to allow for staff adjustments for patient volume and procedures

Produces an audit report of appointments without charges

Patient Management

Maintains insurance and patient balances

Enters patient prospects with identifying codes for referral source and needs. Use the information to measure success and services to offer.

Can set up patients on a formal recall or produce a list of patients who meet user-defined selection criteria for mass recalls

Classifies patients who were served in the hospital only or who are emergency room referrals. Allows for analysis of such patients.

Can store patient pharmacy

Tracks patient treatments and records by case or ailment

Can assign multiple patients to a guarantor

Accommodates at least three insurance companies per patient

Accepts user-defined data items for a patient

Office Routing

Accepts insurance preauthorizations with contact, purpose, procedures, and authorization code

Allows for easy and convenient navigation through the system

Calculates co-pay at time of visit

Allows front desk operator to enter patient information easily at time of visit

Provides checkout desk tools to schedule appointments, enter charges and payments, and produce statements

Accepts payment at time of service

Produces balance sheet by operator for end-of-day reconciliation

Tags transactions with entry date as well as transaction date

Performs close at end of day by employee

Tracks inventory based on procedure code use

Payments

Verifies expected amount when insurance payment comes in

Calculates writeoffs for participating insurance companies

Accepts specific fee schedule for reduced fee arrangements, and bills reduced fee to specific insurer

Attaches notes to EOB or transaction to detail transaction or document issue

Promotes billing to next insurance or to patient after payment

Issues insurance status for payment followup

Holds payment posting until entire payment has been allocated

Submits electronic claims and receives electronic EOBs

Does not split checks on deposit slips

Maintains unapplied payments

Medical Records

Accepts user-defined medical record structure with field definitions

Maintains audit trail and control over changes to medical records

Enters new patient intake information by sex

Can enter prescriptions in system and track refills

Accepts dictated notes by day and provider. Can print notes on label stock for paper records.

Can enter ad hoc note with type (problem, note) and followup action

Accepts scanned images that can be associated with a specific medical record or encounter

Can handle workers' compensation claims

Accepts and stores lab results from outside labs and office lab

Tracks chart location and selects charts for archiving

Managed Care

Can accept patient panel for primary care physician

Can identify patients for preventive medical care

Tracks incoming and outgoing referral authorizations

Verifies fees for incoming referral authorization with fee schedule for plan

Supports capitation plan analysis and patient service requirements

Hospital

Logs patients into hospital

Provides audit tools to track hospital charges for physician as well as outpatient procedures

Associates hospital patient number with hospital stay for transaction matchup on claims

Separates claims requiring surgical notes on claim processing

Accesses hospital computer to review patient information

Collections

Supports collections based on A/R aging with letters and contact management

Manages insurance collection efforts and statuses

Can produce multiple, flexible statement formats

Provides online selection of accounts based on selection criteria

Management Reports

Calculates outstanding services on referral authorizations

Analyzes activity:

- By Modifier
- By Provider
- By ZIP Codes
- By Insurance
- By Provider by Site
- By Age
- By Sex
- By Procedure

APPENDIX 3 • SAMPLE IMPLEMENTATION PLAN

Installation Preparation

1. Depending on the final decision to convert data from the existing system:
   - Review the mapping of information between the new system and the old system to determine data that will have to be modified or adjusted during the conversion process, or
   - Establish a procedure to move the existing accounts to the new system manually.
2. Design any custom forms (e.g., statements), screens (e.g., clinical treatment records), and use of features (e.g., billing groups) to be established during the installation process.
3. Develop an acceptance test for customization of the software, to verify the operation of new capabilities.
4. Design policies and procedures to support operations, take advantage of the investment, and achieve practice objectives. Address the following issues:
   - Patient service
   - Clinical record management
   - System maintenance

     —Business

     —Cycles

     —Scheduling

     —Operations

     —Reporting

Production Schedule Compilation

1. Compile a test suite of data to use during the training process.
2. Establish computer operations, production scheduling, and operational standards to support use of the new system.
3. Review access to power, phone lines, and workspace to accommodate additional terminals and printers.
4. Develop a training schedule.

Installation

1. Install hardware.
2. Convert data electronically or establish schedule to enter current patients manually. Verify data conversion through audit and reconciliation procedures.
3. Train key users on the system and new procedures, including:
   - Software setups
   - Staff-specific procedures
   - Cross-training
   - Super-user issues and responsibilities
4. Train all users on the new system and procedures.
5. Activate system.

Post-Installation

1. Review operations weekly for two months.
2. Review operations monthly thereafter.

APPENDIX 4 • SOFTWARE VENDORS

This Appendix consists primarily of an extensive table compiling the vendor responses to a survey. Vendors were asked to provide information about whether their systems could support the following requirements:

- Scheduling—Can enter provider schedules and assign patients to a schedule slot.
- Patient Treatment—Can enter in several steps to address a problem and track treatments against the plan.
- Managed Care—Can set up outpatient referrals and accept inpatient referrals.
- Medical Records—Accepts several user-defined medical forms or records that can be filled out.
- Collections—Can enter and track patients' promises to pay.
- Electronic Claims—Supports submission of electronic claims to insurers.
- Report Writer—Allows the practice to defined its own reports.
- Accounting—Generates a journal entry to an accounting system to maintain a complete general ledger. (Provide name of accounting system.)

In addition, to obtain a general idea of the cost of each software package, the survey asked vendors to estimate the price of two systems. The systems will be installed at a single location. The estimated price includes basic scheduling, patient billing, insurance billing, and electronic claims capabilities.

1. Vendors were asked to quote a price for a basic practice management system to meet the needs of a two-provider practice with three terminals and two printers. The practice manages 6,000 patients overall and serves 70 patients per day. Hardware, software, and training for four staff members is included in the quote.
2. Vendors were asked to quote a price for a system to meet the needs of a six-provider group that is buying 10 terminals and five printers to serve 12,000 patients overall and handle 150 encounters per day. Hardware, software, training for 12 staff members, and additional costs for medical records software are included in the estimate.

The cost of a system can vary widely depending on the capabilities of the system, the target market, and the number of installations; for this reason, some vendors declined to quote a price. For example, some systems are targeted to specific specialties (e.g., surgery, family practice). Other systems with few installations must spread their costs over a smaller number of users.

The actual cost of a system could also differ dramatically from these estimates depending on the modules purchased and the specific way the practice uses the system. For example, practices that keep patient information online indefinitely may need much more disk space than practices that purge information frequently.

Vendor Product Address Phone Number	Service Area Operating System	Number Installs 1st Install Date	Modules* UD = Under Development							Pricing**		Accting Module
			SCHDL	TREAT	MNGCR	MEDRC	COLLT	ECS	RW	3 User	10 User	
ACC, Inc. **FOXMED WIN** 12500 San Pedro, Suite. 460 San Antonio, TX 78216 210-545-1010 210-545-5545 (fax) E-mail: acc@foxmed.com Website: http://www.foxmed.com	Nationwide Windows 95, Windows NT	6,000 + 1987	X	X	X	X	X	X	X	\$10,000– \$18,000	\$26,000– \$45,000	Quick Books
Advanced Data Systems Corporation **MEDICS II** 255 Spring Valley Avenue Maywood, NJ 07607 800-899-4237 201-368-8377 (fax) E-mail: info@adsc.com Website: http: //www.adsc.com	Nationwide Windows NT, Windows 95	2,600 1977	X	X	X	X	X	X	X	\$10,000 and up	\$25,000 and up	Interfaces Available
American Medical Software **PRACTICE MANAGEMENT PLUS** PO BOX 236 #7 Glen-Ed Prof Park Edwardsville, IL 62025-0236 800-423-8836 618-692-1809 (fax) E-mail: sales@americanmedical.com Website: http://www.americanmedical.com	Nationwide Windows Windows NT	2,100 + 1984	X	X	X	X	X	X	X	**5 User** \$7,995 Software only	**Additional** Users \$1,000 each	**All ASCII**

Artificial Intelligence, Inc. **PAS-3 EASY and PAS-3 PLUS/ AEIC-ELECTRONIC CLAIMS** 354 Upland Drive Seattle, WA 98188 800-533-8902 206-575-2129 (fax) E-mail: artificialintelligence@msn.com Website: http://www.ndex.comai.htm	Nationwide DOS, Windows	4,600 1976	X		X		X	X	X	$1,495– $6,195	$6,495 Does not include hardware	
ASP Software **MEDx** 1031 E. Duane, Suite M Sunnyvale, CA 94086 800-822-7832 408-738-0617 (fax) E-mail: jcoy@compuserve.com	Nationwide DOS, Windows	800 1988	X	X	X	X	X	X	X	$1,490 Software only	$1,490 Software only	Built into software
Axis Clinical Software, Inc. **OUTCOMES MANAGEMENT** 5201 South Westgate Dr., Suite. 216 Portland, OR 97221 800-669-2497 503-291-7392 (fax)	International DOS, Windows, UNIX	N/A (software only)		X	X		X			$25,000 (4 users)	$53,000 (12 users)	
C&S Research Corp. **MEDICAL MANAGEMENT SOLUTION** 1001 W. Ninth St., Suite A King of Prussia, PA 19406 800-545-8460 610-265-0786 (fax) E-mail: info@csrc.com Website: http://www.csrc.com	Nationwide Windows, AIX, UNIX	2000 + 1978	X	X	X	X	X	X	X	$32,000	$58,000	Yes

* **SCHDL** = Scheduling **TREAT** = Treatment Plan **MNGCR** = Managed Care **MEDRC** = Medical Records
COLLT = Collections **ECS** = Electronic Claims Submission **RW** = Report Writer

** 3 User includes hardware, software, and training unless noted. 10 User includes hardware, software, training, and medical records unless noted.

Vendor Product Address Phone Number	Service Area Operating System	Number Installs 1st Install Date	Modules* UD = Under Development							Pricing**		Accting Module
			SCHDL	TREAT	MNGCR	MEDRC	COLLT	ECS	RW	3 User	10 User	
Civitec Healthcare Computers **CIVITEC MEDICAL SYSTEM** 8447 Holly Rd. Grand Blanc, MI 48439 800-949-8016 810-695-9715 (fax) E-mail: civitec@aol.com Website: http://www.civitec.com	Nationwide UNIX, Windows, AIX	1,300 + 1988	X		X	X	X	X	X	$14,500	$38,000	Peachtree Quicken
Clinical Networx Inc. **CLINICAL MASTER** 275 Wyman Street, Suite 210 Waltham, MA 02451 781-890-0888 781-890-8960 (fax) E-mail: sales@cnrx.com Website: http://www.cnrx.com	Nationwide Windows	21 1995	X	X	X	X			X	$7,200 Software only	$19,000 Software only	Can Interface
Clinitec International, Inc. **NEXTGEN** Cedar Creek Corporate Center 195A Witmer Road Horsham, PA 19044 215-957-5490 215-657-7011 (fax) Website: http://www.clinitec.com	Nationwide UNIX, Windows, Novell	77 (current product) 1993			X	X			X	$50,000 Software only	$130,000 Software only	Can interface

Com1 Software, Inc. **C1 SERIES** P.O. Box 482 Hudson, OH 44236 330-653-3771 E-mail: c1soft@aol.com Website: http://www.members.aol.com/c1soft	Nationwide DOS, Windows	2,000 + 1992	U D	X	X	X	X	X	X	Series Model 136	Series Model 136	N/A
CompuSense, Inc. **MEDISENSE** 20 Trafalgar Square Nashua, NH 03063 603-882-6300 603-595-4244 (fax) E-mail: info@compusenseinc.com Website: http://www.compusenseinc.com	Northeast DOS, Windows, Novell	300 + 1990	X		X	X	X	X	X			Available
CompuSystems, Inc. **COMPUSYSTEMS' Medical Practice Management System** 1 Science Court, Carolina Research Park Columbia, SC 29203-9356 800-800-6472 / 803-735-7700 803-735-7711 (fax) Website: http://www.cs.med.com	SC, NC, GA, FL DOS, Windows, Novell, NT, Multi-user DOS	1001 1979	X			X	X	X	X	$19,900 Turnkey (Medical Records Optional)	$35,900 Turnkey (Medical Records Optional)	
Computer Processing Unlimited **MED/FM Medical Financial Mgmt.** **MED/MC Medical Managed Care** 9235 Activity Road #104 San Diego, CA 92126 888-224-4278 619-530-2615 (fax) E-mail: cpu@cgl.com Website: http://www.cpu.cgl.com	Nationwide OS/400	130 1884 FM 1988 MC	X F M	X	X		X	X	X	$48,000	$83,500 (MEDRC not included)	Cust. Interface G/L Interface

* **SCHDL** = Scheduling **TREAT** = Treatment Plan **MNGCR** = Managed Care **MEDRC** = Medical Records
COLLT = Collections **ECS** = Electronic Claims Submission **RW** = Report Writer

** 3 User includes hardware, software, and training unless noted. 10 User includes hardware, software, training, and medical records unless noted.

Vendor **Product** **Address** **Phone Number**	**Service Area** **Operating System**	**Number Installs** **1st Install Date**	**Modules*** **UD = Under Development**							**Pricing****		**Accting Module**
			SCHDL	TREAT	MNGCR	MEDRC	COLLT	ECS	RW	3 User	10 User	
Computer Solutions **MEDWARE** 1055 N. Dixie Highway, Suite. 2 New Smyrna Beach, FL 32168 800-316-4786 904-423-2571 (fax) E-mail: medw@america.com Website: http://www.medware.com	Nationwide DOS, Windows	2,000 + 1989	X		X	UD	X	X	X	$650 Software only	$650 Software only	
Conceptual Systems Corporation **MEDI$TAT** The Georgian Center 730 SOM Center Road Cleveland, OH 44143-2313 800-533-4718 x153 216-646-0449 (fax)	Regional—OH, IN, WV, KY DOS, Windows (DOS Sessions), Novell	650 1982	X		X		X	X		$5,500 Software only	$7,000 Software only	
Conceptual Systems Corporation **CONCEPT** (formerly CYBERMED) The Georgian Center 730 SOM Center Road Cleveland, OH 44143-2313 800-533-4718 x153 216-646-0449 (fax)	Nationwide Windows, Windows 95, Windows NT	50 1995	X	X	X	X	X	X	X	$7,995 Software only	$8,500 Software only	Dynamics by Great Plains and Healthpoint ACS

Control-o-fax Corporation **SPECTRAMED ULTRABILL** 3070 West Airline Highway Waterloo, IA 50704 800-344-7777 319-236-7337 (fax)	Nationwide DOS Windows	4,000 +	X	X	X X	X	X X	X X	X	Each product $15,000		
CSC Healthcare Systems, Inc. **PM 2000** 3535 Grandview Pkwy, Suite. 600 Birmingham, AL 35243 800-541-3920 205-970-8300 (fax) Website: http://www.csc.com/hcs	Southeast UNIX	350	X		X		X	X	X	$25,000	$36,000	Interface w/ RealWorld included
CSS, Inc. **MEDISCAN** 311-C Pomona Drive Greensboro, NC 27407 910-852-0680 910-852-0681 (fax) E-mail: css-inc@worldnet.att.net	Nationwide UNIX, Windows	90 1987	X	X	X	X	X	X	X	$18,000	$22,000	Interface w/ RealWorld
CyCare Systems, Inc. **SPECTRAMED**—SEE HBO & Company/PHYSICIAN OFFICE MANAGER												
DataBreeze-**DATABREEZE HEALTHCARE** Merged with IDX Systems Corp.												

* **SCHDL** = Scheduling **TREAT** = Treatment Plan **MNGCR** = Managed Care **MEDRC** = Medical Records
COLLT = Collections **ECS** = Electronic Claims Submission **RW** = Report Writer

** 3 User includes hardware, software, and training unless noted. 10 User includes hardware, software, training, and medical records unless noted.

Vendor Product Address Phone Number	Service Area Operating System	Number Installs 1st Install Date	Modules* UD = Under Development							Pricing**		Accting Module
			SCHDL	TREAT	MNGCR	MEDRC	COLLT	ECS	RW	3 User	10 User	
Data Strategies, Inc. **COMPUMEDIC** 9645 Granite Ridge Dr., Ste. 230 San Diego, CA 92123 619-514-0300 619-514-0322 (fax) Website: http://www.dsisww.com/dsi.htm	Nationwide DOS, Windows	1,200 1981	X	X	X	X	X	X	X	$9,000	$21,000	DOS/Integrated with own GL and AP Windows/Can interface w/others
Datamedic Corp **DATAMEDIC DM 4000** 20 Oser Avenue Hauppauge, NY 11788 800-446-4021 516-435-1062 (fax) E-mail: haupdcs@aol.com Website: http://www.datamedic.com	Nationwide DOS, OS2	2,500 1973	X			X	X	X	X			
Datamedic Corp **PMstation; CHARTstation** 20 Oser Avenue Hauppauge, NY 11788 800-446-4021 516-435-1062 (fax) E-mail: haupdcs@aol.com Website: http://www.datamedic.com	Nationwide AIX, Windows	2,200 1972	X	X	X	X	X	X	X	Available upon request	Available upon request	Interface

DB Consultants, Inc. **AS/PC WIN** 198 Tabor Road Ottsville, PA 18942 610-847-5065 610-847-2298 (fax) E-mail: dondbc@epix.net Website: http://www.dbconsultants.com	Nationwide DOS, Windows 95	6,000	X	X	X	X	X	X	X	$4,395 Software and training	Varies	Interface
Disc Computer Systems, Inc. **DISC MED** 3055 Old Highway Eight Minneapolis, MN 55418 800-879-3472 612-782-7544 (fax)	Nationwide UNIX, AIX	350 1981	X		X	X	X	X	X	$34,000	$64,200	Part of Disc Med
Docs, Inc. **SOAPWARE** 1443 West Sunset Springdale, AR 72764 800-455-7627 501-756-0283 (fax) E-mail: docsinfo@docs.com Website: http://www.docs.com	Nationwide Windows	300 1993		X	X	X			X			Can interface
Elcomp Systems, Inc. (See Medic Computer Systems, Inc.)												

* **SCHDL** = Scheduling **TREAT** = Treatment Plan **MNGCR** = Managed Care **MEDRC** = Medical Records
COLLT = Collections **ECS** = Electronic Claims Submission **RW** = Report Writer

** 3 User includes hardware, software, and training unless noted. 10 User includes hardware, software, training, and medical records unless noted.

Vendor Product Address Phone Number	Service Area Operating System	Number Installs 1st Install Date	Modules* UD = Under Development							Pricing**		Accting Module
			SCHDL	TREAT	MNGCR	MEDRC	COLLT	ECS	RW	3 User	10 User	
Epic Systems Corporation **EPIC MANAGED CARE SYSTEM/CADENCE APPT. SCHEDULING SYS./EpicCare COMPUTERIZED PATIENT RECORD SYS./RESOLUTE PATIENT ACCOUNTING SYS.** 5301 Tokay Blvd. Madison, WI 53711 608-271-9000 608-271-7237 (fax) Website: http://www.epicsys.com	Nationwide UNIX, VMS, Windows		X	X	X	X	X	X	X			
HBO & Company **PRACTICE 2000** (>25 physicians) 301 Perimeter Center North Atlanta, GA 30346 770-804-2807 770-393-6092 (fax) Website: http://www.hboc.com	Nationwide Windows, UNIX		X	X	X		X	X	X			
HBO & Company—CyCare Business Unit **PHYSICIAN OFFICE MANAGER** 7001 N. Scottsdale Rd., Ste. 1000 Scottsdale, AZ 85253 800-545-2488	Nationwide Windows	1,200 + 1994	X	X	X	X	X	X	X	Pricing based per provider @$3,900 for 1 provider	Pricing based per provider	ODBC interface

Health Care Data Systems **ENTITY** 5703 Enterprise Parkway DeWitt, NY 13214 315-446-7111 315-445-2483 (fax) Website: http://www.hcds.com	Nationwide DOS, Windows	2,000	X		X	X	X	X	X			
Health Data Sciences Corp. (HDS) **ULTICARE Patient Care Info. Sys.** 268 West Hospitality Lane San Bernadino, CA 92408 909-888-3282 909-885-0124 (fax) Website: http://www.hdsc.com 612-851-9696	International UNIX	42 1983		X	X	X			X			
Healthcare Automation **THE HOME HEALTH SOLUTION** 167 Point St., Ste. 3A Providence, RI 02903 401-272-6880 401-272-6883 (fax)	International DOS, UNIX, AIX, Novell Network	275 1982	X	X	X	X	X	X	X			Can interface
HealthCare Communications **MEDIMAC 4.0** 300 S. 68th Street Suite 100 Lincoln, NE 68510 800-888-4344 402-466-9044 (fax) Website: http://www.healthcc.com	International Macintosh 7.1 and up	2,700 1983	X	X	X	X	X	X	X	$10,800–$14,800 Training not included	$24,000–$40,000 Training not included	Integrated

* **SCHDL** = Scheduling **TREAT** = Treatment Plan **MNGCR** = Managed Care **MEDRC** = Medical Records
COLLT = Collections **ECS** = Electronic Claims Submission **RW** = Report Writer

** 3 User includes hardware, software, and training unless noted. 10 User includes hardware, software, training, and medical records unless noted.

Vendor **Product** **Address** **Phone Number**	**Service Area** **Operating System**	**Number Installs** **1st Install Date**	**Modules*** **UD = Under Development**							**Pricing****		**Accting Module**
			SCHDL	TREAT	MNGCR	MEDRC	COLLT	ECS	RW	3 User	10 User	
Healthcare Data **HEALTH PROBE** 5311 Mount Pleasant North Drive Greenwood, IN 46142 317-887-1326 E-mail: hcdi@scican.net Website: http://www.scican.net/~hcdi/	International DOS, Windows	600 1994	X	X	X	X	X	UD		$12,500	$27,500	Quick Books
HUB Computer Medical Systems, Inc. **HUB COMPUTER MEDICAL SOFTWARE** 4221 Indian Springs, NE Albuquerque, NM 87109-1911 505-883-5057 505-889-8867 (fax) E-mail: hubcom@swcp.com Website: http://www.swcp.com/~tanman/	Nationwide DOS, Windows, OS2	130 1989	X	X	X	X			X	$12,500	$32,000	Information is available
IDX Systems Corporation **IDXtendR @ the group practice** (formerly GROUP PRACTICE MANAGEMENT SYSTEM (GPMS)) 1400 Shelburne Rd., P.O. Box 1070 Burlington, VT 05402-1070 802-658-2664 802-660-8161 (fax) Website: http://www.idx.com	Nationwide AIX	600 + 1969	X		X	X	X	X	X			

Infosys, Inc. **MED SYS PRACTICE MANAGEMENT SYSTEM** 2720 River Road, Ste. 141 Des Plaines, IL 60018 800-978-4636 847-925-9421 (fax) E-mail: infosys@infosysusa.com	Nationwide DOS, UNIX, Windows, Macintosh	25 1989	X		X		X	X	U D	$14,360	$28,360	MAS-90 Great Plains
ISYS Group **MR2000** 601 Locust, Ste. 1400 Des Moines, IA 50309 800-434-3004/515-237-6604 515-237-6605 (fax)	Nationwide DOS, UNIX	25 1992		X	X	X			X			
JBS, Inc. **MED2000** 317 Jericho Turnpike Smithtown, NY 11787 800-287-0990 / 516-724-5049 516-724-5049 (fax)	Nationwide Windows 3.11 and Windows 95, Windows NT	300 + 1978	X	X	X	X	X	X	X			
Keystone Medical Systems, Inc. **KMS/PCN HEALTH NETWORK** 3 Lemoyne Drive, Ste. 100 Lemoyne, PA 17043 717-763-1616 717-763-6840 (fax) Website: http://www.keymed.com	Mid-Atlantic, Southeast, Southern CA SCO UNIX, AIX	1,200 1987	X	X	X	X	X	X	X	$14,900	$26,900	RealWorld, general ledger, accts payable, payroll

* **SCHDL** = Scheduling **TREAT** = Treatment Plan **MNGCR** = Managed Care **MEDRC** = Medical Records
COLLT = Collections **ECS** = Electronic Claims Submission **RW** = Report Writer

** 3 User includes hardware, software, and training unless noted. 10 User includes hardware, software, training, and medical records unless noted.

Vendor Product Address Phone Number	Service Area Operating System	Number Installs 1st Install Date	Modules* UD = Under Development							Pricing**		Accting Module
			SCHDL	TREAT	MNGCR	MEDRC	COLLT	ECS	RW	3 User	10 User	
Lytec Systems, Inc. (division of National Data Corp.) **LYTEC MEDICAL SYSTEMS FOR WINDOWS** 7050 Union Park Center, Ste. 390 Midvale, UT 84047 800-735-1991 801-562-0256 (fax) Website: http://www.lytec.com	Nationwide Windows 95' Windows 98'	12,000 + 1989	X		X		X	X	X	$995 Software only	$995 Software only; Multiuser single $695	Quicken, QuickBooks, CYMA, or Lytec
MD/WIN CORP. **CACTUS/MD V7.02** 1300 St. Mary Street, Suite 502 Raleigh, NC 27605 919-833-8999 919-833-8007 (fax) E-mail: pr@cactus.mhs.compuserve.com Website: http://www.mdwincorp.com	NC, SC, VA, TN, MD, DC, WV DOS, Windows	375 1994	X	X		X	X	X	X	$25,400	$68,200	Writes SDF only
Medcomp Systems, Ltd. **DOCS** 3075 Veterans Memorial Hwy Ste. 281 Ronkonkoma, NY 11779 516-467-5401 516-467-6105 (fax)	NY Metro Area DOS, UNIX, Windows, AIX	1,600 1984	X		X	X	X	X	X	$8,500 Software and training only	$10,000 Software and training only	All That

Medic Computer Systems, Inc. **+MEDIC** 8601 Six Fork Road, Ste. 300 Raleigh, NC 27615 919-847-8102 919-846-1555 (fax) Website: http://www.medcmp.com	Nationwide UNIX	11,000 1982	X	X	X	X	X	X	X	$6,400	$11,500	Can Interface
Medical Applications Corporation **AVANTA PRACTICE MGMT. SYS** 6345 Balboa Blvd. #213 Encino, CA 91316 818-708-9700 818-708-3811(fax) Web: www.advantasoft.com	CA, NV, Western US Windows, UNIX	150 1979	X			X	X	X	X	$14,000	$53,000	Yes
Medical Digital Technologies, Inc. **MED-OCCUR** 16360 Roscoe Blvd., Ste. 105 Van Nuys, CA 91406 818-892-4638 818-892-3155 (fax) E-mail: mdt@medoccur.com Website: http://www.medoccur.com	Nationwide UNIX, AIX, AMOS, NTQ3	450 + 1983	X	X	X	X	X	X	X	$12,000	$34,000	Can Interface
Medical Manager Corp. **THE MEDICAL MANAGER** 516 Clyde Ave. Mountain View, CA 94043 415-969-7047/800-222-7701 415-969-0118 (fax) Website: http://www.medicalmanager.com	Nationwide DOS, UNIX, AIX, HP-UX, Windows, Novell	23,600 1981	X		X	X	X	X	X	$19,000	$52,000	

* **SCHDL** = Scheduling **TREAT** = Treatment Plan **MNGCR** = Managed Care **MEDRC** = Medical Records
COLLT = Collections **ECS** = Electronic Claims Submission **RW** = Report Writer

** 3 User includes hardware, software, and training unless noted. 10 User includes hardware, software, training, and medical records unless noted.

Vendor **Product** **Address** **Phone Number**	**Service Area** **Operating System**	**Number Installs** **1st Install Date**	**Modules*** **UD = Under Development**							**Pricing****		**Accting Module**
			SCHDL	TREAT	MNGCR	MEDRC	COLLT	ECS	RW	3 User	10 User	
Medical Office Solutions **MEDASSIST** 2520 Northwest 39th St., Ste. 113 Oklahoma City, OK 73112 800-637-2251	Nationwide DOS (Windows avail. summer 1997)	1,050 1989	X	X	X	X	X	X	X	$16,000	$44,000	
Medical Software Systems, Inc. **OPUS III** 2500 N. Pantano Rd., Ste. 250 Tucson, AZ 85715-3721 800-677-6116 520-733-3939 (fax) Website: http://www.opusiii.com	Nationwide DOS, Windows	65 1981	X	X	X	X	X	X	X			Yes
MedicaLogic, Inc. **LOGICIAN** 20500 NW Evergreen Pkwy Hillsboro, OR 97124 503-531-7000 503-531-7001 (fax) Website: http://www.medicalogic.com	Nationwide DOS, Windows 95, Windows NT, Novell Netware	1,000 1989	X	X		X			X	$6,000 Software only		
MegaWest Systems, Inc. **SUMMIT** 345 Bearcat Drive Salt Lake City, UT 84115 801-565-3737 801-466-7206 (fax) Website: http://www.megawest.com	Nationwide AIX, Windows	420 1980	X	X	X	X	X	X	X	$15,000	$40,000	

Micro Perfect Corporation **DOCTOR PERFECT, MD** **DOCTOR PERFECT, DDS** P.O. Box 500 Oakton, VA 22124 703-716-4678 703-716-1064 (fax) Website: http:\\www.microperfect.com	Worldwide DOS, Windows 95' OS/2, Windows 98' MT	60 1995	X	X	X	X	X		X	$14,500	$36,500	Yes
MicroMed Healthcare Information Systems **MICROMED ENTERPRISE PMS** 3340 Peachtree Rd., Ste. 150 Atlanta, GA 30326 404-467-1500 404-467-0501 (fax) Website: http://www.micromed.com	Nationwide Windows, UNIX	6 (in 100 + practices) 1995	X			X	X	X	X	No set pricing	No set pricing	Yes
National Healthnet Systems **SIMON/MEDITOUCH** 1900 Corporate Blvd., NW Suite 400W Boca Raton, FL 33431 800-416-0012 561-994-0182 (fax) Website: http://www.nhnet.com	Nationwide UNIX	1983	X	X	X	X	X	X	X			Yes
National Medical Systems, Inc. (division of Medic Computer Systems) **MED-1** Westboro Executive Park 110 Turnpike Road Westboro, MA 01581 800-766-1588 / 508-366-1588 508-366-5262 (fax) Website: http://www.medcmp.com	Nationwide Windows (Hewlett-Packard)	1,114 + 1982	X	X	X	X	X	X	X	$30,000 Software and hardware	$100,000 Software and hardware	ACCPAC

* **SCHDL** = Scheduling **TREAT** = Treatment Plan **MNGCR** = Managed Care **MEDRC** = Medical Records
COLLT = Collections **ECS** = Electronic Claims Submission **RW** = Report Writer

** 3 User includes hardware, software, and training unless noted. 10 User includes hardware, software, training, and medical records unless noted.

Vendor Product Address Phone Number	Service Area Operating System	Number Installs 1st Install Date	Modules* UD = Under Development							Pricing**		Accting Module
			SCHDL	TREAT	MNGCR	MEDRC	COLLT	ECS	RW	3 User	10 User	
On Call! Medical Systems **THE ON CALL! MEDICAL SYSTEM** 913 Route 23 South Pompton Plains, NJ 07444 201-839-7100 201-839-6925 (fax)	Metro New York City and New Jersey DOS, Windows, Windows 95	200 + 1992	X		X		X	X	X	$15,000	$29,000	Quicken, Peachtree, One-Write Plus
Patriot Healthcare Development (See Vantage Med)												
Physician Computer Network, Inc. (formerly VERSYSS) **MENDS VERSYSS** 15 Crawford Street Needham Heights, MA 02194 800-899-6400 617-433-0995 (fax) Website: http://www.pcn.com	Nationwide UNIX/AIX 3.25 or later, SCO	7,600 + 1977	X	X	X	X	X	X	X	Varies	Varies	Accounting software
Physician Computer Network, Inc. **PCN HEALTH NETWORK** 1200 The American Road Morris Plains, NJ 07950 800-221-1476 617-433-0995 (fax) Website: http://www.pcn.com	Nationwide SCO UNIX	21,100 1982	X	X	X	X	X	X	X			

Physician Computer Network **SM*RT PRACTICE** 12828 N. Newport Hwy Mead, WA 99021 509-468-7300 509-466-2183 (fax) Website: http://www.wismer.com	Nationwide DOS	1,468 1981	X		X	X	X	X	X			
Physician Micro Systems, Inc. **PRACTICE PARTNER** 2033 Sixth Ave. #707 Seattle, WA 98121 800-770-7674 206-441-8915 (fax) Website: http://www.pmsi.com	Nationwide DOS, UNIX, Novell	2,000 1983	X			X	X	X	X			
Physicians Office Computer **PHYSICIANS OFFICE COMPUTER** 1240 Kona Drive Rancho Dominguez, CA 90220 310-603-0555 310-603-0581 (fax) E-mail: poc@amazingsoftware.com Website: http://www.amazingsoftware.com/poc	Nationwide DOS, Novell, Lantastic NT	3,000 1978	X				X	X		$2,495 Software only		Yes
Physix, Inc. **COMPENDIA/ POCKETCHART** Two Greenway Plaza, Ste. 610 Houston, TX 77046 713-797-1199 713-794-0855 (fax) Website: http://physix.com	Worldwide Windows	2000/ stand-alone and 5 Compendia 1995	X	X		X			X	@ $2,500/user	@ $2,500/user	

* **SCHDL** = Scheduling **TREAT** = Treatment Plan **MNGCR** = Managed Care **MEDRC** = Medical Records
COLLT = Collections **ECS** = Electronic Claims Submission **RW** = Report Writer

** 3 User includes hardware, software, and training unless noted. 10 User includes hardware, software, training, and medical records unless noted.

Vendor Product Address Phone Number	Service Area Operating System	Number Installs 1st Install Date	Modules* UD = Under Development							Pricing**		Accting Module
			SCHDL	TREAT	MNGCR	MEDRC	COLLT	ECS	RW	3 User	10 User	
Q.D. Systems **Q.D. CLINICAL** 2560 9th Street, Ste. 214 Berkeley, CA 94710-2565 800-995-0475 510-705-8865 (fax) Website: http://www.qdsystems.com	International DOS, Windows NT, Novell	2,000 1991	X	X	UD	X			X	$1,995 Software only; stand-alone		
Quality Systems, Inc. **QSI** 17822 East 17th Street Centre Building, Suite 210 Tustin, CA 92780 800-888-7955 / 714-731-7171 714-731-9474 (fax) Website: http://www.qsii.com	Nationwide AIX	535 1977	X	X	X	X	X	X	X			MAS-90
Reynolds and Reynolds Healthcare Systems **KREDO** 9700 SW Nimbus Ave. Beaverton, OR 97008 800-574-5500 503-526-4119 (fax) Website: http://www.reyrey.com	Nationwide UNIX, AS400	100 1993	X		X	X	X	X	X	Starts at $60,000		

Reynolds and Reynolds Healthcare Systems **R/2000** 9700 SW Nimbus Ave. Beaverton, OR 97008 800-574-5500 503-526-4119 (fax) Website: http://www.reyrey.com	Nationwide UNIX, AIX	100 1988	X		X	X	X	X	X	Starts at $60,000		
Scinet **AUTOMATED MEDICAL OFFICE SYSTEM (AMOS)** 11117 Mocking Bird Dr. Omaha, NE 68137 800-736-AMOS 402-331-6660 402-331-8055 (fax) Web: www.scinetinc.com	Nationwide DOS, UNIX, AIX, Netware-Novell	175 1978	X	X	X	X	X	X	X	$15,500	$35,500	MAS-90
SMS **SIGNATURE®** **NOVIUS®** **PHYSICIAN ENTERPRISE MANAGER™** 51 Valley Stream Parkway Malvern, PA 19355 610-219-3378 610-219-8274 (fax) Website: http://www.smed.com	Nationwide IBM-MVS Windows NT	132 1971 1998	X X	 X	X X	 X	X X	X X	X X	N/A	N/A	N/A
Softactics, Inc. **SOFTACTICS MEDICAL BILLING SYSTEM** 1005 Pennsylvania Ave. Ottumwa, IA 52501 515-684-4057 515-682-8976 (fax) E-mail: curtzel@se-iowa.net	Nationwide Multiple User System	75								Varies w/ configurattion	Varies w/ configurattion	

* **SCHDL** = Scheduling **TREAT** = Treatment Plan **MNGCR** = Managed Care **MEDRC** = Medical Records
COLLT = Collections **ECS** = Electronic Claims Submission **RW** = Report Writer

** 3 User includes hardware, software, and training unless noted. 10 User includes hardware, software, training, and medical records unless noted.

Vendor **Product** **Address** **Phone Number**	**Service Area** **Operating System**	**Number Installs** **1st Install Date**	**Modules*** **UD = Under Development**							**Pricing****		**Accting Module**
			SCHDL	TREAT	MNGCR	MEDRC	COLLT	ECS	RW	3 User	10 User	
Sys-Com, Inc. **MEDPAC MEDICAL OFFICE MANAGEMENT SYSTEM** 1218 Oshkosh Ave. Oshkosh, WI 54901 800-543-3767 414-236-4038 (fax)	Nationwide, Bermuda, Bahamas, Puerto Rico DOS	400 + 1986	X	X	X	X	X	X	X	$1,995 Software only; single user	$695 Multi-user upgrade (sets of 4)	ACCPAC PLUS
Systems Plus, Inc.—See Medical Manager Corporation												
Vantage Med **OPTIMIZER/PRACTISMART** 3000 Lake Forest Blvd., Ste. 8 P.O. Box 7049 Tahoe City, CA 96145 888-263-3763 916-583-1532 (fax) E-mail: info@medsoft.com Website:http://www.medsoft.com	Nationwide Windows NT, Windows 95, and Novell	2,000 1985	X	X	X		X	X	X	$1,495 Software only; single user	$2,995 Software only; single user	
VersaForm Corp. **MD VERSAFORM** 591 W. Hamilton Ave. #201 Campbell, CA 95008 800-678-1111 408-370-3393 (fax) E-mail: debra@versaform.com Website: http://www.versaform.com	Nationwide DOS, Windows	4,000 1986	X		X	X	X	X	X	$4,000 Software only	$7,995 Software only	Collection Module

VERSYSS—See Physician Computer Network **MENDS VERSYSS**											
Virtual Software Systems **MEDICAL OFFICE SYSTEM (MOS)** P.O. Box 815 Bethel Park, PA 15102-9417 412-835-9417 412-835-9419 (fax) Website: http://www.vss3.com	Nationwide DOS, UNIX, AIX, LAN, ULTRIX, XENIX, Windows	3,500 1978	X	X	X	X	X	X	X	$14,500 for everything	$30,500 for everything	
Westland Medical Systems **WESTLAND PRACTICE MANAGEMENT SYSTEMS** 23901 Calabasas Road, Ste. 1064 Calabasas, CA 91302 818-591-0081 818-591-7777 (fax)	Western United States UNIX, AIX, HP-UX, SCO UNIX	350 1979	X		X	X	X	X	X	$27,342	$61,418	
WinHealth Systems (division of WindoWare, Inc.) **WINMEDIC!** 219 Windsor Castle Drive, Ste. W Newport News, VA 23608 800-577-9374 / 757-886-0116 719-448-9861 (fax) Website: http://www.pagelink.com	Nationwide Windows	350 1991	X					X		$1,199 Software and training	Network version add $999	Can interface with any Windows product
ZYBEX, Inc. **CYBERMED** 10655 Roselle Street San Diego, CA 92121 619-558-2220 619-558-1537 (fax)	California UNIX, AIX	350 1977	X		X	X	X	X	X	$21,500	$39,000	

* **SCHDL** = Scheduling **TREAT** = Treatment Plan **MNGCR** = Managed Care **MEDRC** = Medical Records
COLLT = Collections **ECS** = Electronic Claims Submission **RW** = Report Writer

** 3 User includes hardware, software, and training unless noted. 10 User includes hardware, software, training, and medical records unless noted.

INDEXES

Subject Index

Name Index

N

O

P

Q

R

S

U

V

W

Z